Dad's Cookbook

Of Family Recipes

William L. Emeny

William L. Emeny, Jr.

Dad's Cookbook
First Edition 2023

S.A.G.E. Publishing

Paperback ISBN: 978-0-9886815-4-5

Dedication

This book is dedicated to Will, Suzy, Mike, their spouses and Sue. It is a labor of love.

.

Contents

Useful Information

Elbows: 1 cup dry weighs 126 grams (4.4 ounces)
1 cup dry elbows cooked 10 minutes weighs 366 grams (12.9 oz); about 2 3/4 cups

Dash salt = 155 gm sodium
1/8 tsp salt = 290 gm
½ tsp salt = 1162 gm sodium

Equivalents Chart

Equivalents Chart;		
Generally used approximations		
	Grams Per	
Teaspoon	5 grams	
Tablespoon	15 grams	3 teaspoons
1/4 Cup	60 grams	4 tablespoons
1/3 Cup	76 grams	5 1/3 ounces
1/2 Cup	114 grams	4 ounces
Cup	227 grams	8 ounces
Pint	454 grams	16 ounces
Quart	908 grams	32 ounces
Liter	1000 grams	35.3 ounces
Liter	1000 grams	2.2 pounds
Ounce	30 grams	2 Tablespoons
Pound	454 grams	1 Pint
1 gram = 1000 mg		

Beverages

Lemonade

Item	Quantity		Directions
			Makes 7 servings; 8 ounces (227g) each
Sugar, White	1	Cup	Add to 2 qt glass measuring cup;
Water, tap	1	Cup	Add to cup; Cook in microwave on hi for 4 min. Stir until clear
Lemon Juice	1	Cup	Add to 2 qt cup
Water, tap	4	Cup	Add to 2 qt cup; mix. Pour over ice

Serving Size 227 grams About 8 oz.Recipe Total Weight 1,626grams About 57.3 oz

Water	Calories	Protein	Fat	Carbs	Fiber	Sugars	Phos*	Pot*	Sodium*
197	115	0	0	30	0	29	3	37	15

* Values are in mg. All others are in grams

Orangeade

Item	Quantity		Directions
			Makes about 8 servings; 8 ounces each
Orange Juice; frozen 12 oz	12	Ounce	Add to 2-quart pitcher
Water, tap	6 1/2	Cup	Add small amount of water and stir until thawed
Sugar, White	1/4	Cup	Add to pitcher; mix until sugar dissolved.
			Add rest of water; mix well. Pour over ice

Serving Size 227 grams....About 8 oz. Recipe Total Weight 1,930 grams About 68.1 oz

Water	Calories	Protein	Fat	Carbs	Fiber	Sugars	Phos*	Pot*	Sodium*
205	82	1	0	20	0	18	24	252	10

* Values are in mg. All others are in grams

Iced Tea, Sweet

Item	Quantity		Directions
			Makes 11 servings, 8 ounces (227g) each
Water, tap	3	Cup	Add to 1 quart pot with lid
			Add 3 tea bags to pot; bring to boil;
			remove from heat; steep for 5 min
Tea, brewed; black	3	Cup	Add brewed tea to 2 quart pitcher
Sugar, White	1/2	Cup	Add to pitcher and stir until sugar dissolved
Lemon Juice	2	Tablespoon	Add to pitcher
Water, tap	4	Cup	Add to pitcher; stir; serve over ice

Comments

If you don't use sugar, or use an artificial sweetener, you will eliminate 9 grams of sugar from one serving

Serving Size 227 grams About 8 oz. Recipe Total Weight 2,499 grams About 88.1 oz.

Water	Calories	Protein	Fat	Carbs	Fiber	Sugars	Phos*	Pot*	Sodium*
217	37	0	0	10	0	9	1	27	9

* Values are in mg. All others are in grams

Breads

Biscuits, baking powder

Item	Quantity		Directions
			Makes 8 biscuits; 2 ounces (60 grams) each
Flour, All Purpose	2	Cup	Add to large bowl
Baking Powder	3	Teaspoon	Add to bowl
Salt, table	1	Teaspoon	Add to bowl; mix very well
Shortening, Crisco	1/4	Cup	Add to bowl; cut in with pastry fork till evenly mixed
Milk; skim	3/4	Cup	Add milk all at once; mix well
			Pam a 5x9 baking dish; Place batter; in dish
			Smooth top with back of spoon
			Bake @ 450 for 14 -20 minutes until top light brown

Serving Size 60 grams About 2.1 oz. Recipe Total Weight 505grams About 17.8 oz

Water	Calories	Protein	Fat	Carbs	Fiber	Sugars	Phos*	Pot*	Sodium*
23	171	4	6	24	1	1	90	66	465

* Values are in mg. All others are in grams

Bread, Italian, bread machine

Item	Quantity		Directions
			Makes about 17 ounces (473g) of dough; enough for a
			Loaf of bread and 6, six inch rolls
Flour, All Purpose	2 1/8	Cup	add to bread machine pan
Salt, table	1/2	Teaspoon	add to pan
Sugar, White	1	Tablespoon	add to pan
Water, tap	3/4	Cup	add to pan
Oil, Canola	1	Tablespoon	add to pan; Put pan in bread machine; close lid
Yeast, baker's, Dry	3/4	Teaspoon	add to yeast cup; set machine to make pizza dough; turn on
			When done, remove dough from pan, cover with flour,
			Knead until dough is dry. Form into a loaf of bread or
			rolls. Let dough rise in a 105*F oven for 90 minutes
			or more.
			Bake bread or rolls @ 350* F for 20 minutes

Comments:

12 ounces (340g) makes 12-inch pizza. 16 ounces (454g) makes a 16-inch pizza. For Sandwich Rolls cut dough into 6 six-inch rolls, let rise in a 105*F oven until good and plump. For bread, form dough into a loaf; let rise in a 105*F oven until good and plump.

To heat oven to 105*F, turn oven on for 1 minute then turn it off

Serving Size 468 grams About 16.5 oz. Recipe Total Weight About 16.8 oz

Water	Calories	Protein	Fat	Carbs	Fiber	Sugars	Phos*	Pot*	Sodium*
206	1,128	28	16	213	8	13	301	308	1,176

* Values are in mg. All others are in grams

Bread and Rolls, Italian, Mixer

Item	Quantity		Directions
			Makes about 1 1/2 pounds of dough; 692 grams
			Recipe for use with a mixer with a dough hook
Yeast, baker's, Dry	2	Teaspoon	Add to mixer bowl
Water, tap	1	Cup	Warm to 105 *F; add to bowl; Dissolve yeast
Salt, table	1/2	Teaspoon	Add to bowl
Oil, Canola	2	Teaspoon	Add to bowl
Flour, All Purpose	2 1/2	Cup	Add to bowl; mix on speed 2, 1 min use dough hook
Flour, All Purpose	1	Cup	Add flour slowly until dough cleans side of bowl
			Knead on speed 2 for two min
			Bread: Form into a loaf about 12 inches by 4 inches
			Rolls: Roll out dough 5 inches by 3/4 inches thick;
			cut into slices 2 inches wide
			Bake rolls and bread at 350 *F for 20 minutes

Comments

Dough to make a one and one half pound loaf of bread or 9 rolls

Serving Size 694 grams About 24.5 oz. Recipe Total Weight About 24.5 oz.

Water	Calories	Protein	Fat	Carbs	Fiber	Sugars	Phos*	Pot*	Sodium*
289	1,698	48	14	337	14	1	523	544	1,202

* Values are in mg. All others are in grams

Bread, White, Bread machine:

Item	Quantity		Directions
			Makes 15 slices, about 2 oz (57g) each
Flour, All Purpose	3 3/4	Cup	Add to breadmaker pan
Salt, table	1	Teaspoon	Add to bread pan
Milk, Dry Instant Non Fat;	2	Tablespoon	Add to bread pan
Butter	2	Tablespoon	Add to bread pan
Sugar, White	1	Tablespoon	Add to bread pan
Water, tap	1 1/2	Cup	Add to bread pan, place pan in bread maker
Yeast, baker's, Dry	1	Teaspoon	Add to yeast dispenser
			Set bread maker to: Basic, Large, Light
			Takes 4 hours to finish

Comments:

Kidney friendly-- Makes a sizable, tall loaf. -- 15 slices, about 58 grams each – 1 slice cut in half is about the same weight as a slice of store sandwich bread.

Serving Size 58 grams**.....**About 2 oz.Recipe Total Weight About 31.2 oz.

Water	Calories	Protein	Fat	Carbs	Fiber	Sugars	Phos*	Pot*	Sodium*
27	131	3	2	25	1	1	41	45	172

* Values are in mg. All others are in grams

Breading Batter:

Item	Quantity		Directions
			Makes a little over 1 cup of batter
Flour, All Purpose	2/3	Cup	Add to 2 cup measure or small bowl
Garlic, Granulated	1	Teaspoon	Add to bowl
Poultry Seasoning, Homemade	1	Teaspoon	Add to bowl
Pepper, Black ground	1/4	Teaspoon	Add to bowl
Water, tap	3/4	Cup	Add to bowl
Salt, table	1/4	Teaspoon	Add to bowl; Stir until smooth

Comments:

Batter is good on Chicken or Fish

Serving Size 30 grams About 1.1 oz. Recipe Total Weight About 9.4 oz

Water	Calories	Protein	Fat	Carbs	Fiber	Sugars	Phos*	Pot*	Sodium*
21	36	1	0	8	0	0	12	17	68

* Values are in mg. All others are in grams

Corn Bread

Item	Quantity		Directions
			Makes about 10 servings, 2 ounces each
Flour, All Purpose	1 1/4	Cup	Add to 4 cup bowl
Cornmeal; yellow	3/4	Cup	Add to bowl
Sugar, White	1/3	Cup	Add to bowl
Baking Powder	2	Teaspoon	Add to bowl
Salt, table	1/8	Teaspoon	Add to bowl; combine
Milk; skim	1	Cup	Add to bowl
Oil, Canola	2	Tablespoon	Add to bowl
Eggs, large	1	Each	Add to bowl; mix well
			Pour into a lightly Pamed 11 x 7 baking dish
			Bake at 400*F for 20-25 minutes till golden brown

Comments:

Oh, so good! It doesn't last long in our house

Serving Size 60 **grams** About 2.1 oz. Recipe Total Weight About 22.8 oz

Water	Calories	Protein	Fat	Carbs	Fiber	Sugars	Phos*	Pot*	Sodium*
27	145	4	3	25	1	7	87	82	137

* Values are in mg. All others are in grams

Muffins

Item	Quantity		Directions
			Makes 1 dozen muffins; 81g each
Flour, All Purpose	2	Cup	Add to sifter
Baking Powder	2	Teaspoon	Add to sifter
Salt, table	1/4	Teaspoon	Add sifter and sift into large mixing bowl
Sugar, White	1	Cup	Add to bowl; mix well.
Butter	1/2	Cup	Add warm butter to bowl; cut in. Set aside
Eggs, large	1	Each	Add to 1 cup measure; beat
Milk; skim	1	Cup	Add milk to beaten egg to make 1 cup
Vanilla extract	1	Teaspoon	Add vanilla to milk and mix
			Add milk to dry ingredients; combine; do not over mix
			Add 1/2 cup of chocolate chips, blueberries or raisins as desired; mix
			fill greased muffin tins 3/4 full
			For cinnamon topping; sprinkle cinnamon on top and spread 1 tsp brown sugar on top
			Bake at 375 °F for 25 minutes

Serving Size 81grams About 2.9 oz. Recipe Total Weight About 30.9 oz.

Water	Calories	Protein	Fat	Carbs	Fiber	Sugars	Phos*	Pot*	Sodium*
29	248	4	9	38	1	20	79	71	229

* Values are in mg. All others are in grams

Nut Biscuits

Item	Quantity		Directions
			Makes 44 slices; 3 1/2 by 1/2 inches about 21g each
Eggs, large	3	Each	Add to large bowl and beat
Sugar, White	1	Cup	Add to bowl slowly and mix
Oil, Canola	3/4	Cup	Add to bowl
Vanilla extract	1	Teaspoon	Add to bowl
Flour, All Purpose	2 3/4	Cup	Add to sifter
Salt, table	1/2	Teaspoon	Add to sifter. Sift and add to bowl
Walnuts Pieces	1/2	Cup	Chop nuts, add to bowl, mix
			Pour into 11 x 7 glass dish: Bake at 350F 20 -25 minutes
			Turn on to cookie sheet, cut into 1/2 inch slices.
			Bake 10 minutes @ 350*F

Comments

Sue's Dad's favorite cookie.

Serving Size 21 grams About 0.7 oz. Recipe Total Weight About 32.7 oz

Water	Calories	Protein	Fat	Carbs	Fiber	Sugars	Phos*	Pot*	Sodium*
	93	4	5	11	0	5	20	19	32

* Values are in mg. All others are in grams

Pizza Dough, bread machine

Item	Quantity		Directions
			Makes about 17 ounces (473g) of dough; enough
			for a 16 inch pizza
Flour, All Purpose	2 1/8	Cup	add to bread machine pan
Salt, table	1/2	Teaspoon	add to pan
Sugar, White	1	Tablespoon	add to pan
Water, tap	3/4	Cup	add to pan
Oil, Canola	1	Tablespoon	add to pan; Put pan in bread machine; close lid
Yeast, baker's, Dry	3/4	Teaspoon	add to yeast cup; set machine to make pizza dough; turn on
			When done, remove from bread maker, cover with flour,
			Knead until dough is dry. Form into pizza shell
			Let shell rise in a 105*F oven for 30 minutes

Comments:

To heat oven to 105*F, turn oven on for 1 minute then turn it off:

12 ounces (340g) of dough makes a 12-inch pizza; 16 ounces (454g) makes a 16-inch pizza,

Serving Size 468 grams…..About 16.5 oz. Recipe Total Weight About 16.8 oz

Water	Calories	Protein	Fat	Carbs	Fiber	Sugars	Phos*	Pot*	Sodium*
206	1,128	28	16	213	8	13	301	308	1,176

* Values are in mg. All others are in grams

Pizza Dough; Mixer

Item	Quantity		Directions
			Makes about 1 1/2 pounds of dough; 692 grams
			Recipe uses a mixer with a dough hook
Yeast, baker's, Dry	2	Teaspoon	Add to mixer bowl
Water, tap	1	Cup	Warm to 105 *F; add to bowl; Dissolve yeast
Salt, table	1/2	Teaspoon	Add to bowl
Oil, Canola	2	Teaspoon	Add to bowl
Flour, All Purpose	2 1/2	Cup	Add to bowl; mix on speed 2, 1 min use dough hook
Flour, All Purpose	1	Cup	Add. flour slowly until dough cleans side of bowl
			Knead on speed 2 for two min
			Pizza;: Roll out on counter to fit cookie sheet or
			lightly oiled pizza pan
			Turn on oven for 1 minute. Let dough rise for 30 minutes
			Let Rise for less time if you want a thinner shell.
			See recipe for pizza

Comments

Dough to make one 16-inch pizza

Serving Size 694 grams About 24.5 oz. Recipe Total Weight About 24.5 oz.

Water	Calories	Protein	Fat	Carbs	Fiber	Sugars	Phos*	Pot*	Sodium*
289	1,698	48	14	337	14	1	523	544	1,202

* Values are in mg. All others are in grams

Rolls, Cinnamon; Bread Machine

Item	Quantity		Directions
			Type Directions Here
			Makes about 12 cinnamon rolls about 3 ounces each
Eggs, large	2	Each	Beat eggs well in a 2 cup measure or bowl
Milk; skim	1/2	Cup	add to beaten eggs
Water, tap	1/4	Cup	Add warm water to eggs, mix and set aside
Flour, All Purpose	3 1/2	Cup	Add to breadmaker pan
Sugar, White	1/4	Cup	Add to pan
Salt, table	1/2	Teaspoon	Add to pan
Butter	4	Tablespoon	Cut into pats, layer into pan
			Pour egg mixture into pan; don not mix; put pan in breadmaker
Yeast, baker's, Dry	1 1/2	Teaspoon	Add yeast to dispenser Set breadmaker for dough; start.
Sugar, Brown	3/4	Cup	Add to 2 cup measure or a small bowl While waiting,
Cinnamon, Ground	2	Teaspoon	Add sugar and mix; set aside
Flour, All Purpose	1/8	Cup	When done, remove dough and knead adding extra flour until not
			sticky. Roll on a floured surface until 9 inches wide by 1/4 inch thick
Butter	4	Tablespoon	Add to small bowl; melt in microwave @ power level 1
			Spread butter then sugar mix evenly on rolled out dough;
			Cut into 1 1/2 inch wide strips; fold in half, roll into a spiral
			Place on greased cookie sheet. Cover and let rise until twice size
			Bake at 350 *F for about 15- 20 minutes until just starting to brown
			Set aside and let cool while making icing
Sugar, powdered	1/2	Cup	Add to 2 cup measure or small bowl
Milk; skim	1	Tablespoon	Add to bowl
Vanilla extract	1/2	Teaspoon	Add to bowl and mix; icing should be runny
			Dribble 1 teaspoon of icing on each roll. Enjoy

Serving Size 85 grams…..About 3 oz . Recipe Total Weight About 38.8 oz

Water	Calories	Protein	Fat	Carbs	Fiber	Sugars	Phos*	Pot*	Sodium*
26	273	5	8	45	1	17	70	85	167

* Values are in mg. All others are in grams

Rolls, Cinnamon; Mixer

Item	Quantity		Directions
			Makes 26 rolls, about 2.3 ounces (66g) each
Milk; skim	3/4	Cup	Place in 2 cup glass measuring cup;
Sugar, White	1/2	Cup	Add to cup
Salt, table	3/4	Teaspoon	Add to cup
Butter	1/2	Cup	Add to cup
			Heat in microwave until butter melted; stir until sugar is dissolved
Water, tap	1/3	Cup	Heat to 105*F, Place in warmed mixer bowl
Yeast, baker's, Dry	4 1/2	Teaspoon	Add to bowl and dissolve
			Cool milk to 105*F, add to bowl,
Eggs, large	2	Each	Beat eggs and Add to bowl
Flour, All Purpose	5	Cup	Add to bowl, 1/2 cup at a time while mixing; Mix at speed 2 for 2 min
Flour, All Purpose	1	Cup	Add flour 1/2 cup at time; Mix until dough cleans sides of bowl;
			Mix for 2 more minutes; Raise in Pamed bowl till double size.
Sugar, Brown	3/4	Cup	Add to 2 cup meaure bowl
Cinnamon, Ground	2	Teaspoon	Add to brown sugar and mix;
Butter	4	Tablespoon	Melt in microwave in small bowl
			Divide dough in half; roll 1/4 inch thick; spread butter and sugar on
			each half: Cut strips 1 1/4 inch wide, fold in half, roll into a spiral
			place on greased cookie sheet. Cover with cloth and let rise until twice size
			Bake at 350 *F for about 15 to 20 min until just starting to brown
			Set aside and let cool while making icing
Sugar, powdered	1/2	Cup	Add to 2 cup measure or small bowl
Milk; skim	1	Tablespoon	Add to bowl
Vanilla extract	1/2	Teaspoon	Add to bowl and mix; icing should be runny
			Dribble 1 teaspoon of icing on each roll

Serving Size(g) 66 About 2.3 oz. Recipe Total Weight 1,598(g) About 56.4 oz.

Water	Calories	Protein	Fat	Carbs	Fiber	Sugars	Phos*	Pot*	Sodium*
19	218	4	6	36	1	11	57	68	130

* Values are in mg. All others are in grams

Condiments

Dressing French

Item	Quantity		Directions
			Makes 4 cups
			Serving size is about 2 tablespoons
Ketchup	1	Cup	Add to 1 qt mixing bowl
Vinegar, Cider	1/2	Cup	Add to bowl
Sweetener, equal, packet	4	Each	Add to bowl
Oregano	1	Teaspoon	Add to bowl
Garlic, Granulated	1	Teaspoon	Add to bowl
Oil, Canola	2	Cup	Add to bowl
Xanthan Gum	1/8	Teaspoon	Add to bowl; thickener is optional
			Beat on hi for 2 min; serve;

Serving Size 30 grams About 1.1 oz . Recipe Total Weight About 29.5 oz

Water	Calories	Protein	Fat	Carbs	Fiber	Sugars	Phos*	Pot*	Sodium*
11	150	0	16	3	0	2	3	33	92

* Values are in mg. All others are in grams

Dressing Italian

Item	Quantity		Directions
			Makes about 2 cups
Vinegar, Cider	1/3	Cup	Add to quart measure
Oil, Canola	1	Cup	Add to measure
Pepper, Black ground	1/4	Teaspoon	Add to measure
Garlic, Granulated	2	Teaspoon	Add to measure
Oregano	1	Teaspoon	Add to measure
Salt, table	1/2	Teaspoon	Add to measure
Xanthan Gum	1/8	Teaspoon	Add to measure; Optional thickener
Sweetener, equal, packet	3	Each	Add to measure; mix on high speed
			with hand mixer for 1 min

Comments:

Use about a tablespoon of dressing on a small salad

Serving Size 15 grams **.....**About 0.5 oz. Recipe Total Weight About 11 oz

Water	Calories	Protein	Fat	Carbs	Fiber	Sugars	Phos*	Pot*	Sodium*
4	96	0	10	1	0	0	2	8	62

*Values are in mg. All others are in grams

Dressing Ranch

Item	Quantity		Directions
			Makes about 2 1/2 cups
			Serving size is about 2 tablespoons
Mayonnaise, regular	1	Cup	Add to bowl
Pickle Juice, sweet	2/3	Cup	Add to bowl
Water, tap	2/3	Cup	Add to bowl
Oil, Canola	1/3	Cup	Add to bowl
Garlic, Granulated	1	Teaspoon	Add to bowl
Sweetener, equal, packet	1	Each	Add to bowl
			Beat on hi; serve

Serving Size 30 grams   About 1.1 oz.   Recipe Total Weight   About 21.4 oz

Water	Calories	Protein	Fat	Carbs	Fiber	Sugars	Phos*	Pot*	Sodium*
16	113	0	12	2	0	1	4	12	104

* Values are in mg. All others are in grams

Dressing Russian

Item	Quantity		Directions
			makes about 1 cup
Miracle Whip	1/2	Cup	Add to bowl
Ketchup	1/2	Cup	Add to bowl
Worcestershire Sauce	1/2	Tablespoon	Add to bowl
Garlic, Granulated	1	Teaspoon	Add to bowl
Sugar, White	1/2	Tablespoon	Add to bowl
Parsley, dried	1/2	Teaspoon	Add to bowl; mix well

Comments

Serving size is about 2 Tablespoons

Serving Size 30 grams   About 1.1 oz.   Recipe Total Weight   About 9.7 oz

Water	Calories	Protein	Fat	Carbs	Fiber	Sugars	Phos*	Pot*	Sodium*
11	55	0	3	7	0	5	19	159	235

* Values are in mg. All others are in grams

Dressing Sweet Italian

Item	Quantity		Directions
			Makes about 4 1/2 cups; about 30 servings
			Serving size; about 2 tablespoon = 30 grams
Vinegar, Cider	2	Cup	Add to 8cup mixing bowl
Sugar, White	1	Cup	Add to bowl
Mustard Seed	1 1/2	Tablespoon	Add to bowl
Turmeric	1 1/2	Teaspoon	Add to bowl
Celery Seed	1 1/2	Teaspoon	Add to bowl
Ginger, Ground	1/2	Teaspoon	Add to bowl
Peppercorns, Black	1	Teaspoon	Add to bowl and mix well.
			Cook on hi in microwave until sugar dissolved.
			Cook for 2 min on power level 5
Vinegar, Cider	1/2	Cup	Add to bowl of warm liquid
Oregano	1	Teaspoon	Add to bowl
Garlic, Granulated	1	Teaspoon	Add to bowl
Oil, Canola	1	Cup	Add to bowl
Xanthan Gum	1/8	Teaspoon	Optional thickener; Add rounded 1/8 tsp to bowl; mix well
			use Xanthan gum sparingly; gets too thick fast
			Chill in refrigerator for 1 hour before serving

Serving Size 30 About 1.1 oz. Recipe Total Weight About 36.8 oz

Water	Calories	Protein	Fat	Carbs	Fiber	Sugars	Phos*	Pot*	Sodium*
16	85	0	6	6	0	6	5	22	4

* Values are in mg. All others are in grams

Gravy Bouillon, Chicken, Beef

Item	Quantity		Directions
			Makes about 1 1/2 cups of gravy; 6 servings, 1/4 cup each
Water, tap	1	Cup	Add to 2 cup glass measure
Soup, bouillon cube	1	Each	Add to measuring cup
Thyme, dried Leaves	1/2	Teaspoon	Add to measuring cup
Marjoram, dried	1/2	Teaspoon	Add to measuring cup
Garlic, Granulated	1/2	Teaspoon	Add to measuring cup
			Microwave for 3 minutes; stir well
Water, tap	1/2	Cup	add to shaker jar
Flour, All Purpose	1 1/2	Tablespoon	add to shaker jar; shake well, add to measuring cup
			microwave on high 1 minute at a time until thick;
			cook on power level 5 for 3 min; add water if needed

Comments:

Serving size about 1/4 cup or 4 tablespoons

Serving Size 60 grams About 2.1 oz. Recipe Total Weight About 13.2 oz.

Water	Calories	Protein	Fat	Carbs	Fiber	Sugars	Phos*	Pot*	Sodium*
57	11	0	0	2	0	0	4	8	9

* Values are in mg. All others are in grams

Ham Glaze

Item	Quantity		Directions
			Makes about 1 1/2 cups
Sugar, Brown	1	Cup	Add to 4 cup measure
Mustard, dry	1	Tablespoon	Add to 4 cup measure
Ginger, Ground	1	Teaspoon	Add to 4 cup measure
Cloves, ground	1/4	Teaspoon	Add to 4 cup measure
Water, tap	1	Cup	Add to 4 cup measure; can use ginger ale
			Heat in microwave until sugar is dissolved

Comments

Add to fried ham; - good in ham gravy - good on baked ham -- Serving Size is about 2 tablespoons when used as a condiment on baked ham

Serving Size 30 grams About 1.1 oz. Recipe Total Weight About 13.8 oz.

Water	Calories	Protein	Fat	Carbs	Fiber	Sugars	Phos*	Pot*	Sodium*
18	45	0	0	11	0	11	5	21	4

* Values are in mg. All others are in grams

Mustard, Hot

Item	Quantity		Directions
			Makes about 2 tablespoons of hot mustard
Mustard, dry	1	Tablespoon	Add to small bowl
Turmeric	1/2	Tablespoon	Add to bowl
Sugar, White	1/4	Teaspoon	Add to bowl; mix
Water, tap	2	Teaspoon	Add to bowl
Oil, Canola	1/4	Teaspoon	Add to bowl; mix well
			Serving size is about 1/2 teaspoon

Comments:

Just a dab on an egg roll is enough, so be careful

Serving Size 3 grams About 0.1 oz. Recipe Total Weight About 0.8 oz

Water	Calories	Protein	Fat	Carbs	Fiber	Sugars	Phos*	Pot*	Sodium*
1	7	0	0	1	0	0	7	16	0

* Values are in mg. All others are in grams

Salsa, from Canned Tomatoes

Item	Quantity		Directions
			Makes 15 servings; 2 tablespoons each; 1 ounce
Tomatoes, diced; can 15oz	1	Can	Chop or coarsely grind. Add to 1 quart glass bowl
Peppers, Jalapeno canned,	1	Ounce	Finely chop 1 oz of peppers, add to bowl
Onion; medium; 30g	1	Ounce	Chop 1 oz onion, add to bowl
Garlic, Granulated	1/4	Teaspoon	Add garlic to bowl
Vinegar, Cider	2	Tablespoon	Add vinegar to bowl
Sugar, White	1/4	Teaspoon	Add sugar to bowl
Cilantro, dried leaf	1/8	Teaspoon	Add cilantro to bowl, mix
			Simmer 5 minutes in microwave on PL10
			Cool and serve

Serving Size 30 grams   About 1.1 oz.   Recipe Total Weight   About 18.1 oz

Water	Calories	Protein	Fat	Carbs	Fiber	Sugars	Phos*	Pot*	Sodium*
27	10	0	0	2	1	1	9	80	74

* Values are in mg. All others are in grams

Sauce, Alfredo

Item	Quantity		Directions
			Makes about 21 ounces (588g);
Butter	1/2	Cup	Place in 4 cup pyrex cup"
			Microwave on power level 7 until melted
Garlic, Granulated	1/4	Teaspoon	Add to cup
Cream, heavy whipping	1 1/2	Cup	Add to cup
Pepper, Black ground	1/8	Teaspoon	Add to cup
Cheese, Romano	1/2	Cup	Add to cup; microwave on Power Level 7, for 8 min

Serving Size 100 grams   About 3.5 oz.   Recipe Total Weight   About 20.7 oz

Water	Calories	Protein	Fat	Carbs	Fiber	Sugars	Phos*	Pot*	Sodium*
44	422	8	43	3	0	2	187	82	417

* Values are in mg. All others are in grams

Sauce, Barbecue Mammoth

Item	Quantity		Directions
			Makes about 1 1/2 quarts
			Condiment Serving size is 2 tablespoons.
Tomatoes, Puree, 28oz can, no salt	1	Can	Add to 8 cup glass bowl
Sugar, White	1/3	Cup	Add to bowl
Molasses	1/4	Cup	Add to bowl
Vinegar, Cider	1/4	Cup	Add to bowl
Mustard, dry	2	Tablespoon	Add to bowl
Cloves, ground	1/8	Teaspoon	Add to bowl
Pepper, Red ground	1/4	Teaspoon	Add to bowl
Smoke, flavor	1/4	Teaspoon	Add to bowl; Stir, cook in microwave 5 min.
			Stir every min

Comments

Use for Beef or Pork Barbecue - Serving size is about 1 tablespoon when used as a condiment

Serving Size 30 grams About 1.1 oz. Recipe Total Weight About 37 oz

Water	Calories	Protein	Fat	Carbs	Fiber	Sugars	Phos*	Pot*	Sodium*
23	26	0	0	6	0	5	13	143	8

* Values are in mg. All others are in grams

Sauce, Barbecue, Smokey

Item	Quantity		Directions
			Makes about 2 cups.
			Condiment Serving size is 2 tablespoons
Tomato Paste (6 oz.)	1	Can	Add 1 can to 2 cup glass measure
Water, tap	1	Cup	Add to 2 cup glass measure
Cloves, ground	1/8	Teaspoon	Add to 2 cup glass measure
Sugar, Brown	1/4	Cup	Add to 2 cup glass measure
Pepper, Red ground	1/4	Teaspoon	Add to 2 cup glass measure
Ginger, Ground	1	Teaspoon	Add to 2 cup glass measure
Vinegar, Cider	2	Tablespoon	Add to 2 cup glass measure
Smoke, flavor	1/2	Teaspoon	Add to 2 cup glass measure, mix
			Cook on hi in microwave for 3 minutes; simmer
			on power level 3 for 3 minutes.

Comments:

Use with beef or pork cooked in crock pot - Makes a good condiment with pot roast

Serving Size 30 grams About 1.1 oz. Recipe Total Weight About 16.9 oz

Water	Calories	Protein	Fat	Carbs	Fiber	Sugars	Phos*	Pot*	Sodium*
25	18	0	0	4	0	4	9	115	8

* Values are in mg. All others are in grams

Sauce, Barbecue, Sweet

Item	Quantity		Directio ns
			Makes about 1 quart;
			Condiment serving size is about 2 tablespoons.
Tomato, Puree, 28oz can, no salt	1	Can	Add 28 oz can puree to 8 cup glass bowl
Sugar, Brown	3/4	Cup	Add to bowl
Basil, dried leaves	1/2	Teaspoon	Add to bowl
Ginger, Ground	1	Teaspoon	Add to bowl
Cloves, ground	1	Teaspoon	Add to bowl
Vinegar, Cider	1/2	Cup	Add to bowl
Pepper, Red ground	1/8	Teaspoon	Add to bowl, mix
			Cook in microwave for 8 min on power level 10;

Comments

Good with beef, pork or chicken

Serving Size 30 grams About 1.1 oz. Recipe Total Weight About 37.2 oz

Water	Calories	Protein	Fat	Carbs	Fiber	Sugars	Phos*	Pot*	Sodium*
24	22	0	0	5	0	4	10	111	8

* Values are in mg. All others are in grams

Sauce, Cocktail

Item	Quantity		Directions
			Makes about 10 servings, 1 ounce (30gm)
			2 tablespoons each.
Ketchup	1	Cup	Add to small bowl
Horseradish, prepared	2	Tablespoon	Add to bowl
Worcestershire Sauce	1	Teaspoon	Add to bowl, mix well

Comments

Not a good choice for a renal diet because of high sodium

Serving Size 30 About 1.1 oz. Recipe Total Weight About 10.9 oz

Water	Calories	Protein	Fat	Carbs	Fiber	Sugars	Phos*	Pot*	Sodium*
21	29	0	0	8	0	6	8	86	260

* Values are in mg. All others are in grams

Sauce, Egg Foo Yung

Item	Quantity		Directions
			About 20 servings, 15 grams each; 1 tablespoon.
Chicken Broth, low sodium	1	Cup	Add to small sauce pan
Soy sauce, tamari	1	Tablespoon	Add to small sauce pan
Sugar, White	2	Teaspoon	Add to small sauce pan
Vinegar, Cider	2	Teaspoon	Add to pan, stir
Cornstarch	2	Tablespoon	Add to pint jar with lid
Water, tap	2	Tablespoon	Add to jar; Shake until flour is mixed.
			Slowly add to sauce pan. Cook on medium heat
			stirring continuously until sauce thickens

Comments:

Serve over Egg Foo Young; Serving size is about 1 tablespoon - This is a **high sodium** condiment so don't use too much

Serving Size 15 **grams** About 0.5 oz. Recipe Total Weight About 11.4 oz

Water	Calories	Protein	Fat	Carbs	Fiber	Sugars	Phos*	Pot*	Sodium*
13	6	0	0	1	0	0	3	12	73

* Values are in mg. All others are in grams

Sauce, General Toas

Item	Quantity		Directions
			makes 14 ounces: almost 2 cups
Cornstarch	1 1/2	Tablespoon	Add to 2 cup glass measure
Ginger, Ground	2	Teaspoon	Add to 2 cup glass measure
Garlic, Minced	1/2	Teaspoon	Add to 2 cup glass measure
Sugar, White	1/4	Cup	Add to 2 cup glass measure
Pepper, Red ground	1/4	Teaspoon	Add to 2 cup glass measure, mix and set aside
Bouillon, Chicken, cube	1	Each	Place in 1 cup glass measure
Water, tap	1	Cup	add to 1 cup measure
			Boil in microwave; about 3 min. Stir until dissolved
Vinegar, Cider	2	Teaspoon	Add to 1 cup measure
Soy Sauce, low sodium	1	Tablespoon	add to 1 cup measure
Wine, table red	1/4	Cup	add to 1 cup measure and stir
			Slowly add to dry ingredients while stirring; mix well
			microwave until thick; about 4 minutes; stir every minute

Comments:

Great for stir fry. - See Pork, General Toas. This is a **high sodium** sauce. So be careful

Serving Size 392 About 13.8 oz. Recipe Total Weight About 13.9 oz

Water	Calories	Protein	Fat	Carbs	Fiber	Sugars	Phos*	Pot*	Sodium*
309	332	3	1	69	1	52	64	240	1,506

* Values are in mg. All others are in grams

Sauce, Horseradish

Item	Quantity		Directions
			Makes enough for 2 roast beef sandwiches
Mayonnaise, regular	4	Tablespoon	Add to 1 cup glass measuring cup or small bowl
Horseradish, prepared	2	Tablespoon	Add to measuring cup; mix well

Comments:

Use 3 tablespoons of sauce for one sandwich. - If I am making a sandwich for myself, I would rather just put mayo on the bread and then add the horseradish after. That way I can get the right amount of horseradish to suit myself.

Serving Size 42 grams About 1.5 oz. Recipe Total Weight About 3 oz

Water	Calories	Protein	Fat	Carbs	Fiber	Sugars	Phos*	Pot*	Sodium*
18	192	0	20	2	0	1	10	42	235

* Values are in mg. All others are in grams

Sauce, Meatloaf

Item	Quantity		Directions
			Makes about 6 servings, about 2 tablespoons each
Ketchup	1/2	Cup	Add to small bowl
Worcestershire Sauce	2	Tablespoon	add to bowl
Thyme, dried Leaves	1/4	Teaspoon	add to bowl
Oregano	1/4	Teaspoon	add to bowl
Pepper, Red ground	1/8	Teaspoon	Add to bowl, mix

Comments:

30 grams is about 2 tablespoons. ---Watch out, this sauce is high in sodium.

Serving Size 30 grams About 1.1 oz. Recipe Total Weight About 6 oz

Water	Calories	Protein	Fat	Carbs	Fiber	Sugars	Phos*	Pot*	Sodium*
21	29	0	0	8	0	6	10	117	295

* Values are in mg. All others are in grams

Sauce, Raisin

Item	Quantity		Directions
			Makes 8 servings, 2.3 ounces (66g) about 4 tablespoons each
Sugar, White	1	Cup	Add to bowl
Cornstarch	2	Tablespoon	Add to bowl; mix well
Water, tap	1	Cup	Add to bowl; mix well
Raisins, seedless	1/2	Cup	Add to bowl; stir
			Cook in microwave; stir every min till thick, then
			Cook for 2 minutes on power level 5.
Lemon Juice	1/2	Tablespoon	Add to bowl, mix well; serve with ham

Comments:

1 serving is about 4 tablespoons. - Goes good with ham.

Serving Size 66 grams About 2.3 oz. Recipe Total Weight About 18.9 oz

Water	Calories	Protein	Fat	Carbs	Fiber	Sugars	Phos*	Pot*	Sodium*
32	131	0	0	34	0	31	9	68	4

* Values are in mg. All others are in grams

Sauce, Soy and Ginger

Item	Quantity		Directions
			Makes 10.8 ounces
Cornstarch	2	Tablespoon	Add to 1 pint glass jar with tight lid.
Garlic, Granulated	1/2	Teaspoon	Add to jar
Sugar, Brown	2	Tablespoon	Add to jar
Ginger, Ground	1	Teaspoon	Add to jar
Pepper, Black ground	1	Teaspoon	Add to jar
Water, tap	1	Cup	Add to jar
Soy Sauce, shoyu, low sodium	2	Tablespoon	Add to jar. Put on lid. Shake until mixed. Set aside for use with meat or vegetables.

Comments:

Good in meat and vegetable dishes. If used as a condiment, cook in microwave until thick.

Serving Size 307 grams About 10.8 oz. Recipe Total Weight About 10.8 oz

Water	Calories	Protein	Fat	Carbs	Fiber	Sugars	Phos*	Pot*	Sodium*
262	164	3	0	38	1	18	66	202	1,099

* Values are in mg. All others are in grams

Sauce, Tarter

Item	Quantity		Directions
			Makes about 1/2 cup; 2 servings
Miracle Whip	4	Tablespoon	Add to 1 cup glass measuring cup or small bowl
Pickle, Bread & Butter	3	Each	Chop pickles slices finely; add to cup and mix well

Comments

Serving sized is 1/4 cup. There is enough for 2 fish sandwiches

Serving Size 41 grams   About 1.4 oz.   Recipe Total Weight   About 2.9 oz

Water	Calories	Protein	Fat	Carbs	Fiber	Sugars	Phos*	Pot*	Sodium*
9	90	0	7	6	0	4	32	250	250

* Values are in mg. All others are in grams

Sauce, Teriyaki

Item	Quantity		Directions
			Makes about 5 cups; serving size is 2 tablespoons
Cornstarch	1 1/2	Teaspoon	Add to 2 cup glass measuring cup
Ginger, Ground	2	Teaspoon	Add to glass cup
Garlic, Granulated	1/2	Teaspoon	Add to glass cup
Sugar, White	1/4	Cup	Add to glass cup; mix and set aside
Bouillon, Chicken, cube	1	Each	Add to 1cup glass measuring cup
Water, tap	1	Cup	Add to 1cup glass measuring cup
			Bring to a boil in microwave, about 3 minutes. Stir until dissolved.
Vinegar, Cider	2	Teaspoon	Add to 1cup glass measuring cup
Wine, table red	1/4	Cup	Add to 1cup glass measuring cup; Stir.
			Slowly add to dry ingredients while stirring; mix well.
			Cook in microwave on high until thick, about 4 minutes; stir every minute
			Use with Teriyaki Beef and Pepper recipe

Comments

Used in Teriyaki Beef and Pepper recipe.

Serving Size 369 grams About 13 oz. Recipe Total Weight About 13 oz

Water	Calories	Protein	Fat	Carbs	Fiber	Sugars	Phos*	Pot*	Sodium*
298	290	1	1	60	1	52	34	160	970

* Values are in mg. All others are in grams

Desserts

Cake, Applesauce

Item	Quantity		Directions
			Makes about 12 servings, 4 ounces each
Butter	1/2	Cup	Add warm butter to large mixing bowl and cream
Sugar, White	2	Cup	Gradually add sugar to bowl; cream with butter
Eggs, large	2	Each	Add to bowl; beat until well mixed
Applesauce, Unsweetened	1 1/2	Cup	Add to bowl, stir until well mixed
Flour, All Purpose	2 1/2	Cup	Add to sifter
Baking Soda	1 1/2	Teaspoon	Add to sifter
Salt, table	1/2	Teaspoon	Add to sifter
Cinnamon, Ground	1	Teaspoon	Add to sifter
Nutmeg	1/2	Teaspoon	Add to sifter
Allspice	1/4	Teaspoon	Add to sifter; sift twice onto wax paper
			Add dry ingredients to bowl a little at a time and mix
Raisins, seedless	1	Cup	Add to bowl and mix
			Lightly grease and flour 13 x 9 x 2 cake pan
			Place batter into pan and spread evenly
			Bake @ 350* for 45 min or until done

Comments:

My favorite cake; nice and moist.

Serving Size 120 grams   About 4.2 oz.   Recipe Total Weight   About 51.3 oz

Water	Calories	Protein	Fat	Carbs	Fiber	Sugars	Phos*	Pot*	Sodium*
39	351	4	9	66	2	44	60	155	330

*Values are in mg. All others are in grams

Cake, Jiffy Chocolate

Item	Quantity		Directions
			Makes 14 pieces, 3 1/2 ounces each
Flour, All Purpose	2	Cup	Add to sifter
Baking Powder	2	Teaspoon	Add to sifter
Baking Soda	1	Teaspoon	Add to sifter
Salt, table	1/2	Teaspoon	Add to sifter; sift into large mixing bowl
Sugar, White	2	Cup	Add to bowl
Cocoa, Hershey's	1	Cup	Add to bowl; mix well
Butter	2/3	Cup	Add to bowl
Water, tap	2	Cup	Bring to boil; Add to bowl; stir till melted
Eggs, large	2	Each	Add to bowl
Vanilla extract	2	Teaspoon	Add to bowl; mix well
			Pour into 9x13* glass baking dish; pam and floured
			Bake at 350*F for 35 minutes or until done

Comments:

Moist cake; easy to make

Serving Size 100 grams About 3.5 oz. Recipe Total Weight About 52.3 oz

Water	Calories	Protein	Fat	Carbs	Fiber	Sugars	Phos*	Pot*	Sodium*
41	273	4	10	44	2	27	87	114	307

* Values are in mg. All others are in grams

Cookie, Chocolate Mint Sugar

Item	Quantity		Directions
			Makes 40 cookies, 1 ounce each
Flour, All Purpose	2 1/4	Cup	Add to sifter
Baking Soda	1	Teaspoon	Add to sifter
Salt, table	1/4	Teaspoon	Add to sifter, sift; set aside
Butter	1	Cup	Soften; Add to mixer bowl or large mixing bowl;
Sugar, White	3/4	Cup	Add to bowl
Sugar, Brown	3/4	Cup	Packed, Add to bowl
Vanilla extract	2	Teaspoon	Add to bowl;
Eggs, large	2	Each	Add to bowl; beat til creamy
Chocolate Chips, Semi sweet	2	Cup	Add 12 oz bag to bowl, mix
			Drop by rounded teaspoon on ungreased cookie pan
			Bake at 375*F for 8 -10 min

Serving Size 25 grams About 0.9 oz. Recipe Total Weight About 43 oz

Water	Calories	Protein	Fat	Carbs	Fiber	Sugars	Phos*	Pot*	Sodium*
3	111	1	6	14	1	9	21	39	72

* Values are in mg. All others are in grams

Cookie, Molasses Spice

Item	Quantity		Directions
			Makes about 33 cookies, 1 ounce each
Shortening, Crisco	1/2	Cup	Add to mixer bowl
Sugar, Brown	1	Cup	Add to bowl & cream
Eggs, large	1	Each	Add to bowl
Molasses	3/4	Cup	Add to bowl, mix well
Flour, All Purpose	2 1/2	Cup	Add to sifter
Cinnamon, Ground	1	Teaspoon	Add to sifter
Cloves, ground	1/4	Teaspoon	Add to sifter
Ginger, Ground	1	Teaspoon	Add to sifter
Baking Powder	2	Teaspoon	Add to sifter
Salt, table	1/8	Teaspoon	Add to sifter, sift, add to bowl, mix well
Raisins, seedless	1/2	Cup	Add to bowl, mix
			Drop by rounded teaspoon on greased cookie sheet
			Flatten with glass with damp cloth over open end
			Bake at 370*F for 8 min

Serving Size 25 grams About 0.9 oz. Recipe Total Weight About 33.5 oz.

Water	Calories	Protein	Fat	Carbs	Fiber	Sugars	Phos*	Pot*	Sodium*
4	96	1	3	17	0	10	21	128	40

* Values are in mg. All others are in grams

Cookie, Suzy's Oatmeal

Item	Quantity		Directions
			Makes about 44 medium cookies, 1 ounce each
Shortening, Crisco	1	Cup	Add to mixer bowl or large bowl
Sugar, Brown	1	Cup	Add to bowl
Sugar, White	1	Cup	Add to bowl; cream till smooth
Eggs, large	2	Each	Add to bowl
Vanilla extract	2	Teaspoon	Add to bowl, beat well
Flour, All Purpose	1 1/2	Cup	Add to sifter
Salt, table	1/2	Teaspoon	Add to sifter
Baking Soda	1	Teaspoon	Add to sifter; sift. Add to bowl, mix
Oats, rolled, dry	3	Cup	Add to bowl and mix
Raisins, seedless	1	Cup	Add to bowl and mix
			Place dough on ungreased cookie pan by teaspoon
			Bake at 350*F for 10-14 min

Serving Size 25 grams About 0.9 oz. Recipe Total Weight About 43.9 oz

Water	Calories	Protein	Fat	Carbs	Fiber	Sugars	Phos*	Pot*	Sodium*
3	108	1	5	15	1	9	31	50	54

* Values are in mg. All others are in grams

Cookie, Pecan Snowball

Item	Quantity		Directions
			Makes about 25 cookies, 1 ounce each
Butter	1	Cup	Add to mixer bowl
Sugar, powdered	1/2	Cup	Add to bowl
Vanilla extract	2	Teaspoon	Add to bowl
Salt, table	1/4	Teaspoon	Add to bowl & cream
Pecans, shelled halves	3/4	Cup	chop fine, Add to bowl, mix
Flour, All Purpose	2 1/4	Cup	Add to bowl, mix
			Shape in 1 inch balls, place on ungreased pan
			Bake at 400*F for 10 -12 min until set, not brown
Sugar, powdered	1/2	Cup	Roll warm balls in sugar

Serving Size 25 grams About 0.9 oz. Recipe Total Weight About 25.1 oz

Water	Calories	Protein	Fat	Carbs	Fiber	Sugars	Phos*	Pot*	Sodium*
3	128	1	8	12	1	4	20	24	72

* Values are in mg. All others are in grams

Cookie, Sugar Soft Raisin

Item	Quantity		Directions
			Makes about 35 cookies, 1 ounce each
Sugar, White	1	Cup	Add to mixer bowl or large bowl
Butter	1/2	Cup	Add to bowl
Shortening, Crisco	1/2	Cup	Add to bowl
Vanilla extract	3	Teaspoon	Add to bowl; cream
Eggs, large	2	Each	Add to bowl, beat till smooth
Flour, All Purpose	2 1/2	Cup	Add to sifter
Baking Powder	2	Teaspoon	Add to sifter
Salt, table	1/8	Teaspoon	Add to sifter
Cinnamon, Ground	2	Teaspoon	Add to sifter; sift; add to bowl while mixing
Raisins, seedless	1	Cup	Add to bowl, mix
			Drop by Tablespoon of lightly greased cookie pan
			Push down with damp cloth on drinking glass
			Bake at 370*F for 8-9 min

Serving Size 25 grams About 0.9 oz. Recipe Total Weight About 35.4 oz

Water	Calories	Protein	Fat	Carbs	Fiber	Sugars	Phos*	Pot*	Sodium*
4	107	1	5	14	0	7	23	41	55

* Values are in mg. All others are in grams

Cookie Sugar

Item	Quantity		Directions
			Makes 25 cookies; 1 ounce each
Sugar, White	1	Cup	Add to mixer bowl
Shortening, Crisco	1/4	Cup	Add to bowl
Butter	1/2	Cup	Add to bowl & cream together
Eggs, large	1	Each	Add to bowl
Vanilla extract	2	Teaspoon	Add to bowl & mix
Flour, All Purpose	2 1/4	Cup	Add to sifter
Baking Powder	1	Teaspoon	Add to sifter
Salt, table	1/4	Teaspoon	Add to sifter; Sift, add to bowl and mix
			Roll out on floured counter top. Cut and place on
			lightly greased (pam) cookie sheet.
			Bake at 350*F for 9-12 min; do not over cook

Serving Size 25 grams About 0.9 oz. Recipe Total Weight About 25.1 oz

Water	Calories	Protein	Fat	Carbs	Fiber	Sugars	Phos*	Pot*	Sodium*
3	112	1	5	15	0	7	19	15	66

* Values are in mg. All others are in grams

Cookie, Chocolate Chip

Item	Quantity		Directions
			Makes 40 cookies, 1 ounce each
Flour, All Purpose	2 1/4	Cup	Add to sifter
Baking Soda	1	Teaspoon	Add to sifter
Salt, table	1/4	Teaspoon	Add to sifter, sift; set aside
Butter	1	Cup	Soften; Add to mixer bowl or large mixing bowl;
Sugar, White	3/4	Cup	Add to bowl
Sugar, Brown	3/4	Cup	Packed, Add to bowl
Vanilla extract	2	Teaspoon	Add to bowl;
Eggs, large	2	Each	Add to bowl; beat til creamy
Chocolate Chips, Semi sweet	2	Cup	Add 12 ounce bag to bowl, mix
			Drop by rounded teaspoon on ungreased cookie pan
			Bake at 375*F for 8 -10 min

Serving Size 25 grams About 0.9 oz. Recipe Total Weight About 43 oz

Water	Calories	Protein	Fat	Carbs	Fiber	Sugars	Phos*	Pot*	Sodium*
3	111	1	6	14	1	9	21	39	72

* Values are in mg. All others are in grams

Cookie, Shortbread

Item	Quantity		Directions
			Makes about 10 cookies, 2 inches square
Flour, All Purpose	2	Cup	Add to medium mixing bowl
Butter	1/2	Cup	Warm to room temperature; Add to bowl, cut in until fine crumbs
Sugar, White	1/2	Cup	Add to bowl, cut in
Vanilla extract	1/2	Tablespoon	Mix in vanilla and knead until smooth
			Press into an ungreased 12 inch pizza pan;
			Pierce all over with a fork; should be about 1/4 inch thick
			Bake at 400 *F for 12 minutes.
			Cut into 2 inch squares with a pizza cutter while still hot in the pan

Comments

Use a flat bottom cup to press dough onto a 23 inch pizza pan.

Serving Size 47 **grams…..**About 1.7 oz. Recipe Total Weight About 16.6 oz.

Water	Calories	Protein	Fat	Carbs	Fiber	Sugars	Phos*	Pot*	Sodium*
5	213	3	9	29	1	10	30	31	74

* Values are in mg. All others are in grams

Frosting, Butter

Item	Quantity		Directions
			Makes enough to frost a two-layer cake
Sugar, powdered	4	Cup	add to small mixing bowl
Butter	6	Tablespoon	soften butter; 1-2 minutes in micro wave at power level 1; add to bowl; beat until smooth
Milk; skim	1/4	Cup	slowly add to bowl while mixing slowly
Vanilla extract	1 1/2	Teaspoon	add to bowl and mix well

Comments:

Makes enough to frost a two-layer cake

Serving Size 633 grams   About 22.3 oz.   Recipe Total Weight   About 22.3 oz

Water	Calories	Protein	Fat	Carbs	Fiber	Sugars	Phos*	Pot*	Sodium*
74	2,518	3	69	483	0	474	83	140	823

* Values are in mg. All others are in grams

Frosting, Cream Cheese

Item	Quantity		Directions
Cheese, Cream, brick	3	Ounce	Warm in microwave, 2min on power level 1 until soft. Add to bowl;
Butter	3	Tablespoon	Warm in microwave, 2min on power level 1 until soft. Add to bowl;
Vanilla extract	1	Teaspoon	Add to bowl
Sugar, powdered	1 1/2	Cup	Add to bowl, mix

Serving Size 312 grams   About 11 oz.   Recipe Total Weight   About 11 oz

Water	Calories	Protein	Fat	Carbs	Fiber	Sugars	Phos*	Pot*	Sodium*
54	1,316	6	64	185	0	180	102	133	548

* Values are in mg. All others are in grams

Fruit Cake, Ma's

Item	Quantity		Directions
Raisins, seedless	3	Cup	1 pound; Add to glass quart measuring cup
Water, tap	1 1/2	Cup	Add to bowl; cook 5 min in microwave on hi
Butter	4	Tablespoon	Add to bowl, mix, cool
Flour, All Purpose	2 1/2	Cup	Put in sifter
Baking Powder	1	Teaspoon	Add to sifter
Baking Soda	1	Teaspoon	Add to sifter
Salt, table	1/4	Teaspoon	Add to sifter
Cinnamon, Ground	1	Teaspoon	Add to sifter
Cloves, ground	1/2	Teaspoon	Add to sifter
Allspice	1/2	Teaspoon	Add to sifter; sift into large bowl
Sugar, White	1 1/2	Cup	Add to bowl; mix
Eggs, large	2	Each	Beat and add to raisins
Walnut, Pieces	1/2	Cup	Add to flour
Fruit, Candied	1	Cup	Add to flour; mix
			Add raisins & eggs; mix well
			Pour into greased and wax paper lined pans
			Bake at 250 for 3 hours; put pan of water in oven

Comments:

A moist and delicious fruit cake. The recipe was my grandmother's. It used to include candied fruit, but I prefer just raisins.

Serving Size 40 grams About 1.4 oz. Recipe Total Weight About 65.8 oz

Water	Calories	Protein	Fat	Carbs	Fiber	Sugars	Phos*	Pot*	Sodium*
13	114	2	2	23	1	17	28	89	69

* Values are in mg. All others are in grams

Fudge, Chocolate

Item	Quantity		Directions
			Makes about 3 pounds
Sugar, White	4	Cup	Add to 2 quart pot
Milk; skim	1 1/3	Cup	Add to pot
Baking Chocolate,	2	Ounce	Add to pot
Cocoa, Hershey's	1/3	Cup	Add to pot
Corn Syrup, Karo	3	Tablespoon	Add to pot
Salt, table	1/4	Teaspoon	Add to pot; mix, cook till 236*F
Butter	4	Tablespoon	Add to pot; cool
Vanilla extract	2	Teaspoon	Add to pot; beat with wood spoon till smooth
			Pour into 8x11 buttered pan; cool 5 min; Cut into 1inch squares

Serving Size 30 grams…..About 1.1 oz. Recipe Total Weight) About 47.4 oz

Water	Calories	Protein	Fat	Carbs	Fiber	Sugars	Phos*	Pot*	Sodium*
7	96	1	2	20	0	19	17	32	27

* Values are in mg. All others are in grams

Fudge, Penuche

Item	Quantity		Directions
			Makes 10 ounces
Sugar, White	1	Cup	Add to 2 qt pan
Milk; skim	2/3	Cup	Add to pan
Corn Syrup, Karo	2	Tablespoon	Add to pan
Molasses	2	Tablespoon	Add to pan
Salt, table	1/4	Teaspoon	Add to pan
			Cook to 234*F on low-medium heat; stir occasionally
Butter	2	Tablespoon	Stir in butter; cool to lukewarm
Vanilla extract	2	Teaspoon	Hand Beat till smooth and starts to change color; pour in 5x8 pan immediately
			Cut into 1 inch squares

Serving Size 30 grams About 1.1 oz. Recipe Total Weight About 17.2 oz

Water	Calories	Protein	Fat	Carbs	Fiber	Sugars	Phos*	Pot*	Sodium*
11	80	0	1	17	0	17	12	56	57

* Values are in mg. All others are in grams

Pie Crust

Item	Quantity		Directi ons
			Makes 0ne 9 inch pie shell
Flour, All Purpose	1	Cup	Add to sifter
Salt, table	1/4	Teaspoon	Add to sifter; sift into large bowl
Shortening, Crisco	1/3	Cup	Add to bowl and cut in
Water, tap	1/4	Cup	Add to bowl; mix and gather into a ball
			Place ball on heavily floured counter top; flatten into an 8 inch round disk.
			Roll out dough until it fits into the pan.
			Perforate crust on bottom and sides of pan every inch or so.
			Bake at 400*F for 7 to 10 min or until crust STARTS to brown. Do not overcook.

Comments:

For best results, handle the dough as little as possible.

Serving Size 252 grams About 8.9 oz. Recipe Total Weight About 9 oz

Water	Calories	Protein	Fat	Carbs	Fiber	Sugars	Phos*	Pot*	Sodium*
73	1,059	13	69	95	3	1	135	133	592

* Values are in mg. All others are in grams

Pie, Apple

Item	Quantity		Directions
			Makes 8 servings, about 7 1/2 ounces (210g) each
Apples, 3" diameter	6	Each	Peel and slice Empire Apples; set aside.
Sugar, White	3/4	Cup	Add to 2 cup measure or small bowl
Flour, All Purpose	3	Tablespoon	Add to bowl
Cinnamon, Ground	1	Teaspoon	Add to bowl
Nutmeg	1/4	Teaspoon	Add to bowl
Allspice	1/4	Teaspoon	Add to bowl and mix well
Pie Crust	1	Each	Place pie crust in 9 inch pie pan.
			Layer apples and sugar mixture on crust
Butter	2	Tablespoon	Layer pats on top of apples
Pie Crust	1	Each	Place top crust and seal to bottom crust with fork
			ventilate 8 or 10 places around top
			Bake @ 400*F for 50 minutes or until the crust starts
			to turn golden brown; do not overcook.

Serving Size 210 grams About 7.4 oz. Recipe Total Weight About 59.3 oz

Water	Calories	Protein	Fat	Carbs	Fiber	Sugars	Phos*	Pot*	Sodium*
124	436	4	20	61	3	31	52	149	173

* Values are in mg. All others are in grams

Pie, Banana Cream

Item	Quantity		Directions
			8 servings, 6 ounces (170g) each
Banana's, Fresh; 7inch	2	Each	Slice bananas and place evenly in pie crust
Vanilla Cream Pudding	1	Each	Pour over sliced bananas in cooked pie shell; let cool

Comments:

To make a banana cream pie, use the vanilla cream pudding recipe and pour it over 2 sliced bananas.

Serving **Size** 170 **grams** About 6 oz. Recipe Total Weight About 48.2 oz

Water	Calories	Protein	Fat	Carbs	Fiber	Sugars	Phos*	Pot*	Sodium*
103	330	7	13	46	1	26	127	249	187

* Values are in mg. All others are in grams

Pie, Chocolate Cream

Ite m	Quantity		Directions
			Makes 12 servings, 4 ounces (120g) each
Eggs, large	3	Each	Beat in 1qt bowl and set aside
Sugar, White	1 1/4	Cup	Add to 8 cup glass bowl
Flour, All Purpose	1/3	Cup	Add to bowl
Cornstarch	2	Tablespoon	Add to bowl
Milk; skim	2	Cup	Slowly add to bowl and mix
Chocolate, unsweetened baking square	2	Ounce	Shave and Add to bowl
			Cook on hi in microwave; stir every min until thick
			Cook on hi for 2 min
			Slowly add to eggs while whisking briskly
			Return mix to 8 cup bowl and microwave 2 min
Butter	2	Tablespoon	Add to bowl and stir until melted
Vanilla extract	1	Teaspoon	Add to bowl and stir
Pie Crust	1	Each	Pour into baked pie shell or dessert cups; chill

Comments:

Optional: Add 1/8 teaspoon of spearmint extract for a chocolate mint pie filling. Mint extracts are not all the same strength, so be careful. Try a small amount then add more if necessary

Serving Size 120 grams About 4.2 oz. Recipe Total Weight About 45.6 oz

Water	Calories	Protein	Fat	Carbs	Fiber	Sugars	Phos*	Pot*	Sodium*
60	299	6	13	41	1	26	112	153	113

* Values are in mg. All others are in grams

Pie, Pumpkin

Item	Quantity		Directions
			Makes 12 servings, 132g (4.7 ounces) each
Pumpkin, Canned	2	Cup	use whole 15 oz can; add to mixer bowl
Sugar, White	3/4	Cup	Add to bowl
Salt, table	1/2	Teaspoon	Add to bowl
Cinnamon, Ground	1 1/4	Teaspoon	Add to bowl
Ginger, Ground	1/2	Teaspoon	Add to bowl
Nutmeg	1/2	Teaspoon	Add to bowl
Cloves, ground	1/4	Teaspoon	Add to bowl; mix
Milk, Evaporated	1 1/2	Cup	Add 12 oz can to bowl
Milk; skim	2/3	Cup	Add to bowl
Eggs, large	3	Each	Add to bowl; blend for 1 min
Pie Crust	1	Each	Pour into unbaked 9 inch crust
			bake at 400F° for 50 min or until knife between center and edge comes out clean

Serving Size 132 grams About 4.7 oz. Recipe Total Weight About 56.3 oz

Water	Calories	Protein	Fat	Carbs	Fiber	Sugars	Phos*	Pot*	Sodium*
88	216	6	9	28	2	18	128	231	206

* Values are in mg. All others are in grams

Pie, Strawberry Glaze

Item	Quantity		Directions
			Makes about 12, four ounce (120 grams) servings
Sugar, White	1	Cup	Add to 1 qt glass mixing bowl
Cornstarch	4	Tablespoon	Add to bowl
Water, tap	1	Cup	Add to bowl slowly and mix well
Strawberries, raw, sliced	2	Cup	Slice strawberries about 1/8 inch thick. Add to bowl
Lemon Juice	1	Tablespoon	Add to bowl
			Microwave on hi, 1 min, stir; repeat until thick
Strawberries, raw, sliced	2	Cup	Place in baked 9 inch pie shell
Pie Crust	1	Each	Pour filling over fruit in pie shell; cool & serve

Comments

If you like strawberries, you will love this pie.

Serving Size 116 grams About 4.1 oz. Recipe Total Weight About 49.5 oz.

Water	Calories	Protein	Fat	Carbs	Fiber	Sugars	Phos*	Pot*	Sodium*
77	181	1	6	31	1	19	25	97	51

* Values are in mg. All others are in grams

Pie, Vanilla Cream

Item	Quantity		Directions
			Makes 1 nine inch pie; 8 servings, 8 ounces (227g) each
Sugar, White	3/4	Cup	Add to 8 cup pyrex dish
Cornstarch	3	Tablespoon	Add to dish
Flour, All Purpose	3	Tablespoon	Add to dish
Salt, table	1/8	Teaspoon	Add to dish and mix well
Milk; skim	2	Cup	Add to dish slowly and mix well
Eggs, large	3	Each	Beat well and set aside
			Stir milk & sugar mixture; Cook in micro wave for 1 minute
			Continue to stir and cook for 1 minute until thick then
			Cook on power level 7 for 2 minutes. Stir well and
			Slowly add hot mixture to eggs while beating vigorously
			Return mixture to 8 cup dish; micro wave, PL 7 for 2 minutes
Butter	2	Tablespoon	Add to dish and stir until melted
Vanilla extract	2	Teaspoon	Add to mixture, stir well;
Pie Crust	1	Each	pour pudding into baked pie shell; let cool and serve

Serving Size 141 grams About 5 oz. Recipe Total Weight About 39.9 oz.

Water	Calories	Protein	Fat	Carbs	Fiber	Sugars	Phos*	Pot*	Sodium*
81	304	6	13	39	1	22	120	144	187

* Values are in mg. All others are in grams

Pudding, Chocolate

Item	Quantity		Directi ons
			Makes 6 servings, about 4 ounces each
Eggs, large	3	Each	Beat in1 quart bowl, set aside
Sugar, White	1 1/4	Cup	Add to 8 cup measuring bowl
Cornstarch	3	Tablespoon	Add to measuring bowl
Milk; skim	2	Cup	Slowly add to measuring bowl and mix
Chocolate, unsweetened baking square	2	Ounce	Shave and add to measuring bowl
			Cook on high in microwave; stir every minute until thick
			Slowly add eggs while whisking briskly
			Cook on high in microwave for 2 minutes.
Butter	2	Tablespoon	Add to bowl, stir until melted
Vanilla extract	1	Teaspoon	Add to bowl and stir
			Divide pudding into 9 desert bowls; chill

Comments:

Very rich and not good for any diet, but oh! so good.. Add 1/8 tsp of spearmint extract to make chocolate mint pudding. Better yet.

Serving Size 114 grams About 4 oz. Recipe Total Weight About 35.5 oz

Water	Calories	Protein	Fat	Carbs	Fiber	Sugars	Phos*	Pot*	Sodium*
65	230	5	8	36	1	32	117	166	70

* Values are in mg. All others are in grams

Pudding, Vanilla

Item	Quantity		Directions
			Makes 8 servings of 4 ounces (112g) each
Eggs, large	2	Each	Add to 4 cup glass measuring cup; beat well; set aside
Sugar, White	3/4	Cup	Add to 8 cup Pyrex cup
Cornstarch	3	Tablespoon	Add to 8 cup Pyrex cup
Salt, table	1/8	Teaspoon	Add to 8 cup Pyrex cup; mix well
Milk; skim	2	Cup	Add to 8 cup Pyrex cup; mix well
			Cook in microwave on HI for 2 min; stir
			Continue to cook for 1 minute and stir until thick then
			Cook on power level 7 for 2 minutes; stir well
			Slowly add to beaten eggs while beating vigorously
			Return mixture to 8 cup Pyrex cup; cook in microwave on power level 7 for 2 minutes
Butter	2	Tablespoon	Add to mixture and stir until melted
Vanilla extract	2	Teaspoon	Add to mixture, mix well; pour into pudding cups or bowl; serve cool

Comments:

This is a very rich and flavorful pudding and a little goes a long way. Add 1/8 teaspoon of spearmint extract for an even better treat.

Serving Size 112 grams.....About 4 oz. Recipe Total Weight About 28.3 oz.

Water	Calories	Protein	Fat	Carbs	Fiber	Sugars	Phos*	Pot*	Sodium*
74	169	4	5	28	0	25	98	129	116

*Values are in mg. All others are in grams

Pudding, Rice

Item	Quantity		Directions
			Makes 10 servings about 3.6 ounces (103g) each
Milk, Evaporated	3/4	Cup	Add 1 can to 8 cup bowl
Milk; skim	1	Cup	Add to bowl
Sugar, White	1	Cup	Add to bowl
Vanilla extract	2	Teaspoon	Add to bowl
Cinnamon, Ground	1	Teaspoon	Add to bowl
Nutmeg	1/2	Teaspoon	Add to bowl; mix well
Rice, White, uncooked	1	Cup	Add to bowl; mix
			cook in microwave on Hi for 3 min
			Cook in microwave on power level 3 until thick and rice tender?

Serving Size 103 grams About 3.6 oz. Recipe Total Weight About 29.4 oz

Water	Calories	Protein	Fat	Carbs	Fiber	Sugars	Phos*	Pot*	Sodium*
48	226	4	2	48	0	29	105	148	39

* Values are in mg. All others are in grams

Sauce, Butterscotch

Item	Quantity		Directions
			Makes 3 1/2 cups; 23 servings of 2 tablespoon each
Sugar, Brown	1	Cup	Add to 2 qt pot
Sugar, White	1/2	Cup	Add to pot
Milk; skim	1/2	Cup	Add to pot
Corn Syrup, Karo	1/4	Cup	Add to pot; Cook on medium heat until a soft ball forms in
			Cool water, 240*F on a candy thermometer; stir often.
			Remove pot from burner.
Butter	4	Tablespoon	Add to pot, stir until melted
Milk, Evaporated	6	Ounce	Add to pot, stir until smooth
Whiskey, 86 proof	1 1/2	Ounce	Add to pot, stir until combined. Enjoy

Comments:

Terrific on vanilla ice cream

Serving Size 30 grams About 1.1 oz. Recipe Total Weight About 25.4 oz.

Water	Calories	Protein	Fat	Carbs	Fiber	Sugars	Phos*	Pot*	Sodium*
12	82	1	2	14	0	14	21	40	32

* Values are in mg. All others are in grams

Sauce, Chocolate

Item	Quantity		Directions
			Makes 33 ounces
Milk, Evaporated	1 1/2	Cup	Add 1 can (12oz) to 2 qt glass measuring bowl.
Sugar, White	2	Cup	Add to bowl
Chocolate, unsweetened baking square	4	Ounce	Shave chocolate, add to bowl. Microwave on hi until chocolate melted. Whisk every minute.
			Remove mixture from heat.
Butter	4	Tablespoon	Add to bowl, stir till melted.
Vanilla extract	1	Teaspoon	Add to bowl, stir; serve warm over ice cream
			Serving size is 2 tablespoons; about 1 ounce (30 g)

Comments:

So much better than chocolate sauces bought in a store.

Serving Size 30 grams About 1.1 oz. Recipe Total Weight About 33.7 oz

Water	Calories	Protein	Fat	Carbs	Fiber	Sugars	Phos*	Pot*	Sodium*
9	101	1	4	15	1	14	39	66	25

* Values are in mg. All others are in grams

Sauce, Strawberry

Item	Quantity		Directions
			makes about 5 servings
Strawberries raw	8	Ounce	Wash 1 quart of strawberries, slice and add to a 2 quart bowl
Vanilla extract	1/2	Teaspoon	Add to bowl
Sugar, White	1/2	Cup	Add to bowl, mix lightly; refrigerate for an hour or more

Comments:

Good on shortcake or ice cream. Can be used with Unjury Protein for a strawberry flavored high protein shake.

Serving Size 60 grams About 2.1 oz. Recipe Total Weight About 11.6 oz.

Water	Calories	Protein	Fat	Carbs	Fiber	Sugars	Phos*	Pot*	Sodium*
38	85	0	0	22	1	20	10	65	1

* Values are in mg. All others are in grams

Shortcake

Item	Quantity		Directions
			Makes 12 servings, 2.1 ounces (60g) each
			Preheat oven to 375*F
Flour, All Purpose	2	Cup	Add to sifter
Baking Powder	3	Teaspoon	Add to sifter
Salt, table	1/4	Teaspoon	Add to sifter; sift into bowl
Sugar, White	1/2	Cup	Add to bowl and mix
Butter	1/2	Cup	Soften butter and add to bowl; cut in with a pastry fork; Set aside.
			To soften butter, warm in microwave for 1 min on power level 1.
Eggs, large	1	Each	Place in 1cup glass measure; beat well
Milk; skim	3/4	Cup	Add milk to eggs to make 1 cup
Vanilla extract	1	Teaspoon	Add to cup measure; mix
			Add egg & milk to bowl, mix slightly; batter is thick and lumpy.
			Place batter in 7 x 9 glass dish lightly sprayed with Pam.
			Batter is thick; spread evenly with spoon.
			Bake @ 375*F for 25 - 30 minutes until golden brown ;serve warm

Comments:

This is heaven with strawberries and whipped cream---This is an old fashion recipe, half way between cake and biscuit.

Serving Size 60 **grams** About 2.1 oz. Recipe Total Weight About 25.3 oz

Water	Calories	Protein	Fat	Carbs	Fiber	Sugars	Phos*	Pot*	Sodium*
21	190	3	8	26	1	9	74	56	246

* Values are in mg. All others are in grams

Shortcake, Strawberry

Item	Quantity		Directions
Shortcake	2	Ounce	Cut shortcake into 3 1/2 X 1 1/2 inch pieces; split in half
Strawberry Sauce	1/4	Cup	Spoon strawberry sauce over shortcake
Whipped Cream, Homemade	1/4	Cup	Top with homemade whipped cream

Comments:

There should be enough shortcake, strawberry sauce and whipped cream for 8 servings using the included recipes for each.

Serving Size 157 grams **About 5.5 oz.** **Recipe Total Weight** **About 5.5 oz.**

Water	Calories	Protein	Fat	Carbs	Fiber	Sugars	Phos*	Pot*	Sodium*
78	435	5	27	45	1	29	108	151	248

* Values are in mg. All others are in grams

Whipped Cream:

Item	Quantity		Directions
			Makes about 6 servings; about 1.3 ounces or 37 grams each
			Put a 2 qt bowl and mixer beaters in freezer for an hour
Cream, heavy whipping	1	Cup	Add cream to cooled bowl; mix on high until cream thickens and starts to peak
Sugar, powdered	2	Tablespoon	Add to bowl
Vanilla extract	1/4	Teaspoon	Add to bowl, mix slightly or until desired thickness
			Be CAREFUL; if you mix too long, it will turn into butter

Serving Size 37 grams About 1.3 oz. Recipe Total Weight About 9 oz

Water	Calories	Protein	Fat	Carbs	Fiber	Sugars	Phos*	Pot*	Sodium*
20	127	1	13	3	0	3	20	33	9

*Values are in mg. All others are in grams

Meats, Soups, Casseroles

Bean Soup

Item	Quantity		Directions
			Makes about 14 cups
Beans, Great Northern, dry	1	Pound	add to 4 quart pot
Water, tap	10	Cup	Add to pot
			Bring to boil; then simmer until soft; 2-3 hours
Ham, roasted	1	Cup	Dice; Add to pot
Sausage, Hot Italian Homemade	1/2	Pound	Crumble and add to pot
Marjoram, dried	1	Teaspoon	Add to pot
Oregano	1	Teaspoon	Add to pot
Pepper, Black ground	1	Teaspoon	Add to pot
Onion; medium; 110g	1/2	Cup	Add 1/2 cup of diced onion to pot

Serving Size 115 grams About 4.1 oz. Recipe Total Weight About 115.5 oz.

Water	Calories	Protein	Fat	Carbs	Fiber	Sugars	Phos*	Pot*	Sodium*
96	83	6	2	10	3	0	99	270	86

* Values are in mg. All others are in grams

Beans, Boston Baked

Item	Quantity		Directions
			Makes about 20 four ounce servings
Beans, Great Northern, dry	1	Pound	Add to 4 quart pot
Water, tap	8	Cups	Add to pot; boil for 15 min; throw off water
Water, tap	6	Cups	Add to pot; boil until beans are soft and liquid thickens; stir often;
			Pour into 11 x 7 baking dish
Sugar, Brown	1/2	Cup	Add to dish
Molasses	1/2	Cup	Add to dish
Bacon, slice, Uncooked	4	Each	cut 4 slices into 1 inch pieces; lay flat on top of beans
			cook in microwave, power level 5, for 30 min
			Or Bake in oven for 45 minutes at 300*F

Comments:

This recipe is high in potassium; be careful. Don't eat too much!

Serving Size 115 grams About 4.1 oz. Recipe Total Weight About 78.6 oz.

Water	Calories	Protein	Fat	Carbs	Fiber	Sugars	Phos*	Pot*	Sodium*
80	142	6	2	25	5	11	117	469	54

* Values are in mg. All others are in grams

Beans, Giacobbi

Item	Quantity		Directions
Beans, Dry Pinto	1	Pound	Add to 4 qt pot
Water, tap	8	Cups	Add to pot, boil for 15 min; throw off water
Water, tap	8	Cup	Add to pot
Ham	1/2	Cup	Dice ham and add to pot
Bacon, slice, Uncooked	4	Each	Finely Chop bacon slices, Add to pot
Pepper, Black ground	3/4	Teaspoon	Add to pot
Salt, table	1/2	Teaspoon	Add to pot
			Boil covered, low heat, until beans are soft; about 2hr

Serving Size 120 grams About 4.2 oz. Recipe Total Weight About 89.4 oz

Water	Calories	Protein	Fat	Carbs	Fiber	Sugars	Phos*	Pot*	Sodium*
97	101	6	3	14	3	0	105	321	144

*Values are in mg. All others are in grams

Beef and Broccoli Stir Fry

Item	Quantity		Directions
			Makes about 5 servings; 9 ounces each
Cornstarch	2	Tablespoon	Add to 1 pint mixing jar with lid
Garlic, Granulated	1/2	Teaspoon	add to jar
Sugar, Brown	2	Tablespoon	add to jar
Ginger, Ground	1	Teaspoon	add to jar;
Water, tap	1	Cup	add to jar
Soy Sauce, low sodium	3	Tablespoon	Add to jar; put lid on jar and shake until well mixed. set aside
Broccolli, frozen,	10	Ounce	Cook in microwave on hi heat for 5 min; drain and set aside
Oil, Canola	2	Tablespoon	Add to large fry pan
Beef, top sirloin, steak	1	Pound	Cut into 1/4 inch thick, 2 inch long strips; add to fry pan
Pepper, Black ground	1	Teaspoon	Add to fry pan
Onion; medium; 110g	1	Each	Peel and cut into 1/4 inch slices; cut slices in half; add to fry pan
			Cook & stir over med-hi heat until beef is done and onion is soft; reduce heat
			Shake cornstarch mixture; add to fry pan; simmer until thick. Stir often
			Simmer and stir for 3 minutes; add water if too thick

Comments:

Serve over rice

Serving Size 246 grams About 8.7 oz. Recipe Total Weight 1,434(g) About 50.6 oz.

Water	Calories	Protein	Fat	Carbs	Fiber	Sugars	Phos*	Pot*	Sodium*
187	302	19	15	22	2	5	211	419	334

*Values are in mg. All others are in grams

Beef and Peppers

Item	Quantity		Directions
			Makes 5 servings; about 8 ounces (217 gram) each
Bouillon Cube, Beef	1	Each	Add 1 cube to 1 cup glass measure
Water, tap	1	Cup	Add to glass cup; cook in microwave on high for 3 min; stir until dissolved
			Add to large fry pan
Mushrooms, white, raw	2	Cup	Mushrooms sliced, Add to fry pan
Peppers, Bell raw, sliced	1	Cup	Slice peppers 1/2 inch wide; 1 inch long; Add to fry pan
Onion; medium; 110g	1	Each	Medium onion sliced thin, Add to fry pan
Beef, Round, raw	1/2	Pound	Slice thin and cut 1 inch long. Add to fry pan
Pepper, Black ground	1/4	Teaspoon	Add to fry pan
Ginger, Ground	1	Teaspoon	Add to fry pan
Worcestershire Sauce	1	Tablespoon	Add to fry pan
Sugar, White	1	Tablespoon	Add to fry pan
Basil, dried leaves	1	Teaspoon	Add to fry pan; mix
			Cover pan; Simmer 6 min on medium heat
Cornstarch	2	Tablespoon	Add to shaker jar
Water, tap	1	Cup	Add to shaker jar; shake well
			Slowly add to fry pan; stir constantly
			Stir constantly until thick; add water if necessary

Comments:

Serve with rice or egg noodles

Serving Size 218 grams About 7.7 oz. Recipe Total Weight About 38.6 oz

Water	Calories	Protein	Fat	Carbs	Fiber	Sugars	Phos*	Pot*	Sodium*
189	134	11	6	10	1	5	130	348	264

* Values are in mg. All others are in grams

Beef Roast

Item	Quantity		Directions
			Makes about 12, four-ounce (120 grams) servings
Beef, Round, raw	3	Pound	Place in glass baking dish
Thyme, dried Leaves	1	Teaspoon	Spread on beef and bottom of pan
Marjoram, dried	1	Teaspoon	Spread on beef and bottom of pan
Pepper, Black ground	1/4	Teaspoon	Spread on beef and bottom of pan
Garlic, Granulated	1/2	Teaspoon	Spread on beef and bottom of pan
Parsley, dried	1	Teaspoon	Spread on beef and bottom of pan
			Cook in 325* oven to 150*F, about 3 hrs
			To make gravy: Put meat on a platter and then
			Pour liquid from pot roast pan into 4 cup measure;
			To make gravy, follow separate recipe for roast beef gravy

Comments:

Makes great sandwiches with some mayo and horseradish; -- see recipe for roast beef sandwich

Serving Size 120 grams About 4.2 oz. Recipe Total Weight About 48.2 oz

Water	Calories	Protein	Fat	Carbs	Fiber	Sugars	Phos*	Pot*	Sodium*
78	234	25	14	0	0	0	239	414	65

* Values are in mg. All others are in grams

Beef Roast with Gravy

Item	Quantity		Directions
			Makes about 12, four ounce (120 grams) servings of beef
			Makes about 17 ounces of gravy; about 12 1.5oz servings
Beef, Round, raw	3	Pound	Place in glass baking dish
Thyme, dried Leaves	1	Teaspoon	Spread on beef and bottom of pan
Marjoram, dried	1	Teaspoon	Spread on beef and bottom of pan
Pepper, Black ground	1/4	Teaspoon	Spread on beef and bottom of pan
Garlic, Granulated	1/2	Teaspoon	Spread on beef and bottom of pan
Parsley, dried	1	Teaspoon	Spread on beef and bottom of pan
			Cook in 325* oven to 150*F, about 3 hours
			When cooked, put meat on a platter; pour liquid from pan
			into a 4 cup measure.
Water, tap	2	Cup	Add water to make 3 cups; add to fry pan, stir,
Flour, All Purpose	4	Tablespoon	Add flour to pint shaker jar with lid;
Water, tap	1	Cup	Add to shaker jar and shake till all flour is mixed
			Wisk flour mixture into fry pan, mix well;
Thyme, dried Leaves	1/2	Teaspoon	Add to fry pan
Marjoram, dried	1/2	Teaspoon	Add to fry pan; mix well
			Cook on medium heat; stir constantly until thick;
			Simmer for 2 minutes; Add water or flour water needed

Comments:

3 tablespoons of gravy are about 1.5 ounces (45gm); A dash of salt is 155 milligrams of sodium

Serving Size 156 grams About 5.5 oz. Recipe Total About 74.4 oz

Water	Calories	Protein	Fat	Carbs	Fiber	Sugars	Phos*	Pot*	Sodium*
119	206	21	12	2	0	0	204	352	57

* Values are in mg. All others are in grams

Beef Stew

Item	Quantity		Directions
			Makes8 servings, 8ounce (226 gram) each
Beef, Chuck	1 1/2	Pound	Cut into 3/4 inch cubes; place in crock pot
Water, tap	1/2	Cup	Add to pot
Potatoes, white	8	Ounce	Peel 3 small potatoes, cut in half; add to pot
Onion; medium; 110g	1/2	Each	2 to 2 1/2 inch onion; Slice 1/4 thick; Add to pot
Mushrooms, white, raw	4	Ounce	Slice 6 medium mushrooms, add to pot.
Thyme, dried Leaves	1/2	Teaspoon	Add to pot
Marjoram, dried	1/2	Teaspoon	Add to pot
Parsley, dried	1/2	Teaspoon	Add to pot
Peppers, Bell, raw chopped	4	Ounce	Dice,1 medium pepper; Add to pot
Garlic, Minced	1/2	Teaspoon	Add to pot;
Pepper, Black ground	1/2	Teaspoon	Add to pot; Cook on LO for 6-8 hours
			When stew is cooked, pour liquid into a 1 qt Pyrex cup
Water, tap	1	Cup	Add water to cup to make 2 cups of broth; Set aside
Flour, All Purpose	5	Tablespoon	Add flour to shaking jar (16 ounce jar with a lid)
Salt, table	1/8	Teaspoon	Add 1/8 teaspoon salt to to shaking jar
Water, tap	1	Cup	Add water to shaking jar; tighten lid and shake until flour is dissolved
			Add to Pyrex cup. Cook in microwave for 1 minute on HI
			Mix well, Repeat until thick. Add water if too thick.
			Cook for 3 minutes on power level 5; Return gravy to pot or serve separately

Comments:

A Medium onion is 2-2½ inches in diameter and weighs about 110 gm. Good with rice or egg noodles. Good on biscuits except for the extra salt.

Serving Size 226 grams About 8 oz. Recipe Total Weight About 64.4 oz

Water	Calories	Protein	Fat	Carbs	Fiber	Sugars	Phos*	Pot*	Sodium*
185	208	18	10	11	1	1	192	444	110

* Values are in mg. All others are in grams

Beef, Vegetables, Soy-Ginger Sauce

Item	Quantity		Directions
			Makes about 6 servings; 10.7 ounces each
Vegetables, frozen, Asian	10	Ounce	Cook in microwave for 4 minutes on PL 10. Drain, set aside
Oil, Canola	2	Tablespoon	Add to fry pan
Beef, top sirloin, steak,	1	Pound	Cut into 1/8 inch thick strips 2 inches long. Add to fry pan
			Cook and stir over medium heat until beef is done.
			Add cooked vegetables to frypan.
Sauce, Soy and Ginger	37	Ounce	Shake jar of sauce and add to fry pan. Simmer until thick.
			Stir often. Simmer and stir for 2 minutes. Add water if needed.

Comments:

Serve with rice. Recipe is **high in sodium**. Be careful.

Serving Size 303 About 10.7 oz. **Recipe Total Weight About 64 oz.**

Water	Calories	Protein	Fat	Carbs	Fiber	Sugars	Phos*	Pot*	Sodium*
238	320	19	15	28	3	10	207	455	689

* Values are in mg. All others are in grams

Chicken Soup

Item	Quantity		Directions
			Makes2 servings, about 1 cup each
Chicken Broth, low sodium	1	Cup	Add to 2 qt pot
Pepper, Black ground	1/4	Teaspoon	Add to pot
Poultry Seasoning, Homemade		Teaspoon	add to pot
Garlic, Granulated	1/8	Teaspoon	Add to pot
Celery Seed	1/8	Teaspoon	Add to pot
Chicken, Breast, no skin	6	Ounce	Slice ¼ inch thick, 1 inch long
			Simmer until chicken is cooked

Comments:

Serve with rice or ditalini.

Serving Size 205 About 7.2 oz. Recipe Total Weight About 14.5 oz.

Water	Calories	Protein	Fat	Carbs	Fiber	Sugars	Phos*	Pot*	Sodium*
181	102	19	3	1	0	0	192	393	424

* Values are in mg. All others are in grams

Chicken Stir Fry; General Toas

Item	Quantity		Directions
			Makes about 4 servings, 9 ounces (262gm) each
			Prepare recipe for Gen Toas Sauce; set aside
Chicken, Breast, no skin	1	Pound	Slice 1/4 thick; then cut into 1 inch squares; set aside
Onion; medium; 110g	1	Each	Slice 1/4 thick; cut slices in half; set aside
Peppers, Bell, raw chopped	1/2	Cup	Slice into ¼ inch strips; set aside
Celery, raw, cup chopped	1/2	Cup	Chop 1 large (11-12) stalk 1/4 inch thick; cut in half; set aside
Vegetables, frozen, mixed	5	Ounce	Thaw 1/2 10 oz package of oriental veggies; set aside
Oil, Canola	2	Tablespoon	Add to large fry pan; place over medium heat
			Add chicken to pan; sauté on medium heat until chicken is cooked; push aside
Oil, Canola	1	Tablespoon	Add to bare part of fry pan
			Add Onions, peppers, celery and mixed veggies to fry pan; Sauté for 5 minutes
Gen Toas Sauce	1	Cup	Add to fry pan; simmer for 5 minutes on medium heat. Serve over rice

Serving Size 262 grams About 9.2 oz. Recipe Total Weight About 38.5 oz.

Water	Calories	Protein	Fat	Carbs	Fiber	Sugars	Phos*	Pot*	Sodium*
204	289	24	13	18	2	9	259	566	419

* Values are in mg. All others are in grams

Chicken Vegetables and Gravy

Item	Quantity		Directions
			Makes about 12 servings; 1 cup each
Bouillon, Chicken, cube	2	Each	Add to 2 cup glass measure
Water, tap	2	Cup	Add to cup; microwave until cube disolved; about 4 minutes Set Aside
Chicken, Breast, no skin	2	Pound	Slice into 1/4 inch strips; cut strips to 1 inch; add to large fry pan
Oil, Canola	2	Tablespoon	Add to fry pan; cook chicken; all liquid should be gone;
Poultry Seasoning,	2	Teaspoon	Sprinkle evenly on chicken
Pepper, Black ground	1/2	Teaspoon	Sprinkle evenly on chicken, Stir until well mixed
			Add bouillon to pan;
Corn, frozen	10	Ounce	Add 1 10 oz bag Birds eye super sweet corn to pan
Peas, Frozen	10	Ounce	Add 1 10 oz bag Birds eye baby peas to pan
			Simmer until veggies are tender
Water, tap	2	Cup	Add to pan
Flour, All Purpose	4	Tablespoon	Add flour to shaker jar
Water, tap	1	Cup	Add to shaker jar; shake until all mixed
			Bring pan to simmer; shake flour mixture. Slowly add to pan; stir where added
			Simmer until thick; Simmer for 3 minutes; stir constantly; serve

Comments:

Serve on biscuits, toast, rice or egg noodles. Good dialysis recipe; low, phosphorus, potassium and sodium.

Serving Size 227 About 8 oz. Recipe Total Weight About 96.3 oz

Water	Calories	Protein	Fat	Carbs	Fiber	Sugars	Phos*	Pot*	Sodium*
191	159	18	5	12	2	2	196	361	320

* Values are in mg. All others are in grams

Chile, made with Canned Beans

Item	Quantity		Directions
			Makes about 10 servings; about 1 cup each
Tomato Paste (6 oz. can)	2	Can	Add to 4-quart pot
Water, tap	1 1/2	Cup	Add 2 tomato paste cans of water. Wisk until combined
Beans, Kidney 15.5 oz can	2	Can	Add to pot undrained
Beef, Ground 80%; raw	1	Pound	Crumble and add to 4 quart pot
Onion; medium; 110g	1	Each	Dice medium onion, add to pot
Garlic, Granulated	2	Teaspoon	add to pot
Pepper, Red ground	1/2	Teaspoon	add to pot
Cumin	1	Teaspoon	add to pot
Oregano	1	Teaspoon	add to pot
			Bring to boil; Simmer 20 minutes; serve

Comments:

High in potassium, **be careful**: ---Serve with rice or cornbread

Serving Size(g) 212 About 7.5 oz. Recipe Total Weight 2,148(g) About 75.8 oz

Water	Calories	Protein	Fat	Carbs	Fiber	Sugars	Phos*	Pot*	Sodium*
165	219	14	10	21	5	6	198	717	274

* Values are in mg. All others are in grams

Egg Foo Yung

Item	Quantity		Directions
			Makes about 4 servings, 146 grams each
Pork, Shoulder, raw	1/2	Cup	Slice very thin; cook in microwave on power level 5 until done; set aside.
Eggs, large	6	Each	Add to 4 quart bowl, beat lightly
			Add to 4 quart bowl
Mung beans, mature seeds, sprouted, raw	1	Cup	Add fresh bean sprouts to bowl of eggs
Onions, spring or scallions, chopped	1/4	Cup	Add scallions to bowl of eggs
Celery, raw, cup chopped	1/4	Cup	Add celery to bowl of eggs
Soy sauce, tamari	1	Teaspoon	Add soy to bowl of eggs and mix
Oil, Canola	1	Tablespoon	Heat oil in small fry pan on medium heat
			Stir and add 1/3 cup egg mixture to pan and fry as you would a pancake until lightly brown on bottom, turn and brown.

Comments:

Keep warm (but do not stack) while you fry remaining pancakes, add more oil if needed and stir egg mixture before adding to pan. Serve with Hot Egg Foo Young Sauce.

Serving Size 146 grams About 5.1 oz. Recipe Total Weight About 20.7 oz.

Water	Calories	Protein	Fat	Carbs	Fiber	Sugars	Phos*	Pot*	Sodium*
112	201	15	14	3	1	2	221	268	214

*Values are in mg. All others are in grams

Eggs, Omelet, Cheese and Pepperoni:

Item	Quantity		Directions
			Makes 2 servings about 5 ounces each.
Eggs, large	4	Each	Beat 4 eggs in a small bowl
Cream, heavy whipping	4	Teaspoon	Add to bowl
Pepper, Black ground	1/8	Teaspoon	Add to bowl
Garlic, Granulated	1/8	Teaspoon	Add to bowl
Pepperoni, Sliced	8	Each	Cut pepperoni into small pieces, add to bowl.
Cheese, Cheddar shredded	1/4	Cup	Add to bowl
Butter, salted, pat	1	Each	Add 1 pat to 8
			Pour egg mixture into hot fry pan, cook for 6 minutes or until egg starts to get solid on top.
			Fold over and cook for 2 min; serve hot.

Comments:

Cook times will vary with burner temperature and are meant as a suggestion only.

Serving Size 135 grams About 4.8 oz. Recipe Total Weight About 9.5 oz

Water	Calories	Protein	Fat	Carbs	Fiber	Sugars	Phos*	Pot*	Sodium*
90	293	18	24	2	0	1	282	185	380

*Values are in mg. All others are in grams

Eggs, Omelet, Pepperoni

Item	Quantity		Directions
			Makes1 serving of 5.2 ounces (147g) each
Eggs, large	2	Each	Whisk in bowl
Cream, heavy whipping	1	Tablespoon	Add to bowl and whisk
Pepper, Black ground	1/8	Teaspoon	Add to bowl and whisk
Garlic, Granulated	1/8	Teaspoon	Add to bowl and whisk
Onions, raw	2	Tablespoon	Dice Onion, set aside
Pepperoni, Sliced	3	Each	Dice, set aside
Butter, salted, pat	1	Each	Add a pat of butter to fry pan
			Melt butter in fry pan over medium low heat. When butter melts, pour egg mixture into pan.
			Evenly distribute onion, pepperoni over the egg.
			When egg becomes firm, fold over in half
			Cook for 30 seconds; Serve while hot

Comments:

You can use garlic powder instead of granulated garlic, but not garlic salt. --

Serving Size 147 grams About 5.2 oz. Recipe Total Weight About 5.2 oz.

Water	Calories	Protein	Fat	Carbs	Fiber	Sugars	Phos*	Pot*	Sodium*
105	271	15	22	4	0	2	228	209	278

*Values are in mg. All others are in grams

Eggs, Scrambled with Pepperoni

Item	Quantity		Directions
			2 eggs scrambled. 3 diced pepperoni slices. Serves 1
Eggs, large	2	Each	Put in a cup or small bowl; beat slightly
Cream, heavy whipping	1	Teaspoon	Add to cup/bowl; Mix vigorously with a whisk
Pepperoni, Sliced	3	Each	Dice, add to cup
Butter, salted, pat	1	Each	Melt butter in fry pan, Pour egg mixture into heated fry pan
			Cook until eggs begin to set, stir with spatula until desired doneness.

Serving Size 116 grams About 4.1 oz Recipe Total Weight About 4.1 oz.

Water	Calories	Protein	Fat	Carbs	Fiber	Sugars	Phos*	Pot*	Sodium*
82	226	14	18	1	0	1	213	162	273

* Values are in mg. All others are in grams

Fish, Baked Haddock

Item	Quantity		Directions
			Makes two small servings, about 4.5 ounces each.
Fish, Haddock, raw	8	Ounce	Place in glass baking dish
Butter	1	Tablespoon	Melt butter; spread evenly on fish
Garlic, Granulated	1/8	Teaspoon	Spread evenly on fish
Pepper, Black ground	1/8	Teaspoon	Add pepper to taste; Spread evenly on fish
Oregano	1/8	Teaspoon	Spread evenly on fish
Lemon Juice	1	Tablespoon	Spread evenly on fish
			Bake at 350*F for 35 minutes: or microwave 2 minutes at power level 5

Comments:

The garlic, pepper, oregano and lemon juice can be mixed with the melted butter and the combination spread evenly on the fish.

Serving Size 128 grams About 4.5 oz. Recipe Total Weight About 9.1 oz

Water	Calories	Protein	Fat	Carbs	Fiber	Sugars	Phos*	Pot*	Sodium*
102	137	19	6	1	0	0	260	340	288

* Values are in mg. All others are in grams

Fried Rice, Ham and Sausage:

Item	Quantity		Directions
			Makes about 7 servings, 8 ounces (277g) each
Rice, White, long grain	1	Cup	Add to 2 quart sauce pan
Water, tap	2	Cup	Add to pan and cover, bring to boil
			Simmer on low heat for 14 minutes or until water is gone; set aside
Sausage, Hot Italian	12	Ounce	Add to large fry pan; cook and crumble
Ham	6	Ounce	Dice and add to fry pan
Onions, raw, chopped	8	Tablespoon	Dice onion and add to pan
Mushrooms, white, raw	4	Ounce	Dice 6 medium mushrooms, add to pan
Garlic, Granulated	1	Teaspoon	Add to pan
Pepper, Black ground	1/4	Teaspoon	Add to pan;
Corn, frozen	1	Cup	Add to pan
Peas, Frozen	1	Cup	Add to pan
Water, tap	1/4	Cup	Add to pan
Soy Sauce, low sodium	2	Teaspoon	Add to pan; stir; simmer
Eggs, large	1	Each	Beat egg and add to pan; stir
			Simmer until vegies are tender
			Add cooked rice and cook on low heat for 5 min. serve

Serving Size 227 grams About 8 oz. Recipe Total Weight About 62.1 oz.

Water	Calories	Protein	Fat	Carbs	Fiber	Sugars	Phos*	Pot*	Sodium*
169	280	17	11	28	2	2	226	402	452

*Values are in mg. All others are in grams

Fried Rice, Mexican

Item	Quantity		Directions
			Makes 8 servings; 95 gm (3.4 ounces) each
Rice, White, long grain	1	Cup	Add to 1 qt pot
Water, tap	2	Cup	Add to pot; bring to boil; simmer 14 min;
Butter	2	Tablespoon	Add butter to large fry pan and melt; add cooked rice
Peas, Frozen	1/4	Cup	Add to fry pan
Corn, frozen	1/4	Cup	Add to fry pan
Chili Powder, Homemade	2	Teaspoon	Add to pan
Cilantro, dried leaf	1	Teaspoon	Add to pan
Pepper, Red ground	1/8	Teaspoon	Add to pan; cook on med hi; stir a lot

Comments:

This is a side dish, only 2 grams of protein.

Serving Size 95 grams About 3.4 oz. Recipe Total Weight About 26.8 oz

Water	Calories	Protein	Fat	Carbs	Fiber	Sugars	Phos*	Pot*	Sodium*
69	120	2	3	21	1	0	37	58	33

* Values are in mg. All others are in grams

Goulash

Item	Quantity		Directions
			Makes about 6 servings of 2 cups; 260 grams each
			Boil 1 cup of elbows in 4 quart pot for 10 min. Drain & set aside.
Beef, Ground 80%; raw	1	Pound	Cook in large fry pan; spoon out grease when done
Water, tap	1	Cup	Place in glass measuring cup
Bouillon Cube, Beef	1	Each	Add to water in cup
			Bring to boil in microwave, stir till dissolved; set aside
Onion; medium; 110g	8	Tablespoon	dice; add to fry pan when meat is done
Mushrooms, white, raw	1	Cup	Slice; add to fry pan
Garlic, Granulated	1	Teaspoon	Add to fry pan
Thyme, dried Leaves	1	Teaspoon	Add to fry pan
Basil, dried leaves	1	Teaspoon	Add to fry pan
Fennel seed	1/4	Teaspoon	Add to fry pan
Corn, frozen	1/2	Cup	Add to fry pan
Peppers, Bell, raw	1/4	Cup	Dice, add to fry pan
			Add bullion to fry pan, simmer for 5 miutes.
Elbows, cooked	4	Cup	Add cooked elbows; stir, cook 4 minutes.
Worcestershire Sauce	1/4	Cup	Add to fry pan; mix and serve

Serving Size 260 grams About 9.2 oz . Recipe Total Weight About 53.1 oz.

Water	Calories	Protein	Fat	Carbs	Fiber	Sugars	Phos*	Pot*	Sodium*
188	366	20	17	34	2	3	212	462	373

* Values are in mg. All others are in grams

Goulash, Italian

Item	Quantity		Directions
			Makes 6 servings; 220 gm (7.8oz) each
Elbows, cooked	1	Cup	Boil elbows in sauce pan for 10 minutes; drain, set aside
Beef, Ground 80%; raw	1	Pound	Add to large fry pan; cook, crumble, remove fat
Spaghetti sauce with meat	2	Cup	Add to fry pan when beef is cooked; mix well
Onions, raw, cup, chopped	1/2	Cup	Dice onion and add to fry pan
Garlic, Granulated	1	Teaspoon	Add to fry pan
Pepper, Black ground	1/2	Teaspoon	Add to fry pan
Oregano	1	Teaspoon	Add to large fry pan; mix will; simmer until onions soft
			Add cooked elbows, break up lumps and mix well
Mozzarella, shredded, part skim	1	Cup	Sprinkle on top of goulash; continue simmering until melted; serve

Serving Size 220 grams About 7.8 oz. Recipe Total Weight About 44.3 oz

Water	Calories	Protein	Fat	Carbs	Fiber	Sugars	Phos*	Pot*	Sodium*
155	361	23	22	17	2	5	302	624	218

* Values are in mg. All others are in grams

Green Beans, Herbed

Item	Quantity		Directions
			Makes about 3 servings of 3 ounces each
Beans, Green, frozen	8	Ounce	Add to large dish with cover
Marjoram, dried	1/2	Teaspoon	Add to dish
Sugar, White	2	Tablespoon	Add to dish
Butter	2	Tablespoon	Add to dish
Vinegar, Cider	1	Tablespoon	Add to dish
Garlic, Granulated	1/4	Teaspoon	Add to dish
Ginger, Ground	1/2	Teaspoon	Add to dish; cover; microwave 5 min on high

Serving Size 90 grams   About 3.2 oz.   Recipe Total Weight   About 10.5 oz

Water	Calories	Protein	Fat	Carbs	Fiber	Sugars	Phos*	Pot*	Sodium*
67	117	2	7	13	2	9	33	176	58

* Values are in mg. All others are in grams

Ham and Cabbage

Item	Quantity		Directions
			Makes 4 servings; about 5.6 ounces (160 g) each
Potatoes, white	8	Ounce	Peel 1/2 pound of potatoes; cut into 1/2 inch slices; layer into 4 quart pot
Ham, cured	12	Ounce	Cut ham into 1/2 inch thick slices; layer into pot.
Cabbage, raw	2	Pound	Cut a medium head of cabbage into 3/4 inch slices; add to pot
Fennel seed	1/4	Teaspoon	Add ground fennel to pot.
Water, tap	1	Quart	Add to pot.
			Bring water to boil; reduce heat and simmer for 45 minutes. Serve.

Serving Size 160 grams About 5.6 oz. Recipe Total Weight About 85.5 oz.

Water	Calories	Protein	Fat	Carbs	Fiber	Sugars	Phos*	Pot*	Sodium*
144	64	5	2	7	2	2	75	219	302

* Values are in mg. All others are in grams

Hamburg and Vegetables with Gravy

Item	Quantity		Directions
			Makes about 4 servings; 8 ounces (240 gm) each
Beef, Ground 80%;	1	Pound	Add to large fry pan, crumble and cook
Corn, frozen	1	Cup	Add to large fry pan
Onions	1/2	Cup	Dice onion and add to pan
Peppers, Bell,	1/2	Cup	Dice and add to pan
Water, tap	1	Cup	Use Pyrex measuring cup
Bouillon Cube, Beef	1	Each	Add to pyrex cup; microwave on hi for 4 min; stir add to fry pan
Thyme, dried	1	Teaspoon	Add to fry pan
Marjoram, dried	1	Teaspoon	Add to fry pan
Parsley, dried	1	Teaspoon	Add to fry pan
Garlic, Granulated	1	Teaspoon	Add to fry pan
Pepper, Black ground	1/2	Teaspoon	Add to fry pan
Fennel seed	1/4	Teaspoon	Add ground fennel seed to fry pan
			Simmer for 6 to 8 min until pepper is cooked
Water, tap	1	Cup	Add to fry pan , mix
Flour, All Purpose	3	Tablespoon	Add flour to shaker jar
Water, tap	1	Cup	Add to shaker jar; shake until flour dissolved;
			Slowly add to fry pan while stirring briskly; simmer 3 minutes until thick

Comments:

Serve over egg noodles, rice or pasta; Remember, don't cook them in salted water.

Serving Size 240 grams About 8.5 oz. Recipe Total Weight About 52.7 oz

Water	Calories	Protein	Fat	Carbs	Fiber	Sugars	Phos*	Pot*	Sodium*
198	237	14	15	11	1	2	153	321	206

* Values are in mg. All others are in grams

Hamburg and Gravy

Item	Quantity		Directions
			Makes about 6 servings; with 4 ounces (117 gm) of meat each. Plus 2 tablespoons of gravy
Beef, Ground 80%;	8	Ounce	Crumble & Cook in 10 inch fry pan until done
Water, tap	1 1/2	Cup	Add to fry pan and stir.
Pepper, Black ground	1/2	Teaspoon	Add to fry pan
Thyme, dried Leaves	1	Teaspoon	Add to fry pan
Garlic, Granulated	1	Teaspoon	Add to fry pan
Salt, table	1/4	Teaspoon	Add to fry pan and stir
Flour, All Purpose	3	Tablespoon	Add flour to pint jar with top
Water, tap	1	Cup	Add water to jar, Cover jar, shake until flour is all mixed.
			Slowly add to fry pan whisking constantly. Simmer 5 minutes. Add water if necessary.

Comments:

Good over egg noodles or rice. Good on toast or biscuits but they add extra salt-- Don't forget. Do not cook rice or noodles in salted water. Serving size includes 2 tablespoons of gravy.

Serving Size 141 grams About 5 oz. Recipe Total Weight About 30 oz

Water	Calories	Protein	Fat	Carbs	Fiber	Sugars	Phos*	Pot*	Sodium*
122	113	7	8	4	0	0	67	116	128

* Values are in mg. All others are in grams

Hamburg, Zucchini, and Sauce

Item	Quantity		Directions
			Makes about 5, 9 ounce servings
			Start cooking pasta, rice or noodles
Zucchini, raw	2	Cup	Cut medium (8 inch) zucchini into 1/4 inch slices; add to glass dish with a cover.
Onion; medium; 110g	1	Each	Cut medium onion into 1/4 inch slices; add to dish.
Mushrooms, white, raw	4	Ounce	Cut mushrooms into 1/4 inch slices, add to dish.
			Microwave veggies in covered dish for 6 minutes, set aside.
Beef, ground, 85%	12	Ounce	Crumble into a large fry pan; fry until done.
Sauce, Spaghetti,	16	Ounce	Add to fry pan.
Water, tap	1/2	Cup	Add water to fry pan.
			Add zucchini, onion and mushrooms to pan;
			Simmer on low heat for about 5 minutes; serve

Comments:

Serve with egg noodles, rice or pasta. 1 cup of this recipe = 247gm

Serving Size 196 grams   About 6.9 oz.   Recipe Total Weight   About 48 oz

Water	Calories	Protein	Fat	Carbs	Fiber	Sugars	Phos*	Pot*	Sodium*
164	166	13	9	8	2	5	152	558	62

* Values are in mg. All others are in grams

Lasagna

Item	Quantity		Directions
			Makes two 10x14 dishes; about 30 servings (3x3)
Meatballs, Italian	2	Pound	Use recipe for meatballs, crumble and add to large fry pan
Sausage, Hot Italian Homemade	1	Pound	Add to large fry pan; crumble & cook till done; set aside
Lasagna Noodles	1	Pound	Boil 18 in large pot 10 min, nudge often; drain
Cheese, Ricotta, part skim	2	Pound	Add to large bowl\n
Eggs, large	2	Each	Add to large bowl
Parsley, dried	1	Tablespoon	Add to large bowl
Oregano	1	Tablespoon	Add to large bowl
Basil, dried leaves	1	Tablespoon	Add to large bowl; mix well.
			Lightly spray bottom of large glass (10x14) baking dish with Pam
Sauce, Spaghetti, with meat	1/2	Cup	Spread sauce on bottom of dish.
			Place 3 cooked & drained noodles on sauce.
			Spread 1/2 of cheese mix on noodles
			Spread 1/4 of meat mix on cheese mix
Spaghetti Sauce	1/2	Cup	Spread sauce on next. Place 3 noodles next.
Spaghetti Sauce	1/2	Cup	Spread sauce on noodles
Cheese, Mozzarella, sliced,	6	Each	layer mozzarella cheese on sauce
Spaghetti Sauce	1/2	Cup	layer 3 noodles; spread sauce on top
			Layer 1/4 of meat mixture
Spaghetti Sauce	1/2	Cup	Layer sauce
			Bake in 350 degrees*F oven; until 160*F, 1 hour

Serving Size 180 grams About 6.3 oz. Recipe Total Weight About 127.2 oz.

Water	Calories	Protein	Fat	Carbs	Fiber	Sugars	Phos*	Pot*	Sodium*
110	366	23	18	27	2	3	329	430	268

* Values are in mg. All others are in grams

Macaroni and Cheese

Item	Quantity		Directions
			Makes 8 servings, 6 ounces (170g) each
Elbows, cooked	2	Cup	Boil DRY elbows for 10 min in 4 qt pan; drain and set aside
Sausage, Hot Italian Homemade	8	Ounce	Break apart and fry; set aside
Butter	3	Tablespoon	Add to 8 cup glass bowl; melt in microwave; 1min
Flour, All Purpose	3	Tablespoon	Wisk into melted butter
Pepper, Black ground	1/4	Teaspoon	Add to bowl
Fennel seed	1/4	Teaspoon	Grind and add to bowl. Mix well with whisk.
Milk; skim	1 1/2	Cup	Add very slowly to bowl and whisk until smooth
			Cook in microwave on hi until thick; whisk every minute
Cheese, Cheddar, brick	1	Pound	Slice cheese thin and add to bowl.
Cheese, Mozzarella, shredded, part skim	1/2	Cup	Add to bowl; cook on high in microwave until cheese melts;
			Stir every minute. Add cooked sausage to bowl; mix.
			Add cooked elbows and stir
			Cook in microwave for 10 min; serve

Comments:

Mac and cheese is high in phosphorous and sodium and is not a very good choice for a kidney diet; so plan carefully.

Serving Size 170 grams   About 6 oz.   Recipe Total Weight   About 49.8 oz

Water	Calories	Protein	Fat	Carbs	Fiber	Sugars	Phos*	Pot*	Sodium*
100	413	22	29	16	1	3	402	228	496

* Values are in mg. All others are in grams

Meatballs, Italian

Item	Quantity		Directions
			Makes about 34 meatballs which are about 35g cooked
Beef, Ground 80%;	2	Pound	Place into a large bowl
Bread Crumbs, dry	1 1/2	Cup	Add to bowl
Eggs, large	2	Each	Beat and Add to bowl
Cheese, Romano	1/2	Cup	Add to bowl
Parsley, dried	1/4	Cup	Add to bowl
Onions, raw,	1/4	Cup	Chop and add to bowl
Oregano	1	Tablespoon	Add to bowl
Pepper, Black ground	1	Teaspoon	Add to bowl
Water, tap	1/2	Cup	Add to bowl, Mix
			Place meatballs on greased cookie sheet
			Bake in 400*F oven till 150*F; about 20 min

Comments:

Use an ice cream scoop with a lever to release the molded meatballs. Push the meatball mix into the scoop to compact it and keep the meatball together.

Serving Size 140 grams About 4.9 oz. Recipe Total Weight About 51.4 oz

Water	Calories	Protein	Fat	Carbs	Fiber	Sugars	Phos*	Pot*	Sodium*
81	345	22	22	13	1	1	271	321	345

* Values are in mg. All others are in grams

Meatloaf

Item	Quantity		Directions
			Makes 6 3/4 inch, 4 ounce (120g) slices
Beef, Ground 80%; raw	1	Pound	Add to large bowl
Cornmeal; yellow	1/2	Cup	Add to bowl
Bread Crumbs, dry	1/2	Cup	Add to bowl
Ketchup	1/3	Cup	Add to bowl
Eggs, large	1	Each	Add to bowl
Garlic, Granulated	1	Teaspoon	Add to bowl
Basil, dried leaves	1	Teaspoon	Add to bowl
Thyme, dried Leaves	1	Teaspoon	Add to bowl
Parsley, dried	1	Teaspoon	Add to bowl
Water, tap	1/2	Cup	Add to bowl and mix; place in 8.5 x 4.5 x 2.5 glass loaf pan. Cover with plastic wrap
			Cook in microwave; Power level 4 until 160 degrees F; about 15-20 min
			See recipe for Meatball Sauce

Comments:

Serve with meatloaf sauce. Meatloaf sauce is good with a SMALL baked potato.

Serving Size 120 grams About 4.2 oz. Recipe Total Weight About 29.4 oz.

Water	Calories	Protein	Fat	Carbs	Fiber	Sugars	Phos*	Pot*	Sodium*
73	254	14	15	17	1	3	158	275	233

* Values are in mg. All others are in grams

Mushroom Stew

Item	Quantity		Directions
			Makes about 8 servings; 8 ounces each
Mushrooms, white,	8	Ounce	Cut mushrooms into 4 slices; add to glass covered dish.
Zucchini	8	Ounce	Slice Zucchini into 1/4 inch slices; cut into quarters; add to dish.
Onion; medium; 110g	1	Each	Cut onion into 1/4 inch slices; cut in half; add to dish.
			Cover dish, cook in microwave for 6 min; set aside
Beef, Ground 80%	1	Pound	Crumble and Fry in large fry pan
Spaghetti sauce with meat	2	Cup	Add to fry pan
Italian Sausage Seasoning	1/2	Tablespoon	Add to fry pan
Water, tap	1 1/2	Cup	Add to fry pan; heat until simmering Add veggies to fry
			Pan. Simmer for 9 minutes or done to taste.

Comments:

Serve over rice, pasta or egg noodles

Serving Size 120 grams   About 4.2 oz.   Recipe Total Weight   About 65.6 oz.

Water	Calories	Protein	Fat	Carbs	Fiber	Sugars	Phos*	Pot*	Sodium*
101	105	7	7	4	1	2	85	299	51

* Values are in mg. All others are in grams

Oatmeal and Maple Syrup

Item	Quantity		Directions
QUAKER, QuickOats.	1/2	Cup	Pour in deep microwaveable bowl.
Water, tap	1	Cup	Add to bowl. Microwave on high for about 1 minute.
Syrup, Maple	3	Teaspoon	Pour syrup over cooked oatmeal and stir. Enjoy!

Comments:

Makes 1 serving. Microwaves timings vary. You may have to adjust the time up or down.

Serving Size 294 grams About 10.4 oz. Recipe Total Weight About 10.5 oz

Water	Calories	Protein	Fat	Carbs	Fiber	Sugars	Phos*	Pot*	Sodium*
244	199	6	3	40	4	13	183	186	16

* Values are in mg. All others are in grams

Pancakes

Item	Quantity		Directions
			Makes 9 pancakes, about 2 ounces (60g) each
Flour, All Purpose	1 1/4	Cup	Place flour in 1 quart measure cup or bowl
Baking Powder	1	Tablespoon	Add to bowl
Sugar, White	2	Tablespoon	Add to bowl
Salt, table	1/4	Teaspoon	Add to bowl, mix dry ingredients
Eggs, large	1	Each	Place in small bowl, beat until frothy
Milk; skim	1	Cup	Add to bowl of eggs
Vanilla extract	1/4	Teaspoon	Add to bowl of eggs
Oil, Canola	2	Tablespoon	Add to bowl of eggs, mix well
			Add eggs and milk to dry ingredients; mix till almost smooth
			Add 1/4 cup to medium hot fry pan.
			Fry until bubbles appear on top; flip and fry golden brown

Comments:

Fry in medium hot pan PL 6-7. Pan is hot when sprinkle of water sputters. Batter is very thick; smooth over with spoon after adding to pan.

Serving Size 60 grams About 2.1 oz. Recipe Total Weight About 18.3 oz

Water	Calories	Protein	Fat	Carbs	Fiber	Sugars	Phos*	Pot*	Sodium*
32	124	4	4	19	0	4	94	72	257

* Values are in mg. All others are in grams

Pancakes, Sourdough

Item	Quantity		Directions
			Makes 6 pancakes; about 4 ounces (120g) each
Flour, All Purpose	1	Cup	Add to 4 cup bowl
Sugar, White	1	Tablespoon	Add to bowl
Salt, table	1/4	Teaspoon	Add to bowl
Baking Soda	2	Teaspoon	Add to bowl, mix
Milk; skim	3/4	Cup	Add to bowl, mix
Eggs, large	1	Each	Beat egg till fluffy, add to bowl, mix
Oil, Canola	1	Tablespoon	Add to bowl
Sourdough Starter	1/2	Cup	Add to bowl, mix. Fry on 350* griddle.
Milk; skim	1/2	Cup	Add to starter
Flour, All Purpose	1/2	Cup	Add to starter, mix; let sit at room temperature until liquid forms on top;

Serving Size 120 grams About 4.2 oz. Recipe Total Weight About 23.3 oz.

Water	Calories	Protein	Fat	Carbs	Fiber	Sugars	Phos*	Pot*	Sodium*
70	197	7	1	38	1	9	118	145	603

* Values are in mg. All others are in grams

Pancakes, Cornmeal

Item	Quantity		Directions
			Makes 8 pancakes; about 2 1/4 ounces (65g) each.
Cornmeal; yellow	1	Cup	Add to 1qt bowl.
Flour, All Purpose	1/2	Cup	Add to bowl.
Baking Soda	2	Teaspoon	Add to bowl.
Sugar, White	2	Tablespoon	Add to bowl and mix.
Eggs, large	1	Each	Place in 2 cup measuring cup; beat well.
Milk; skim	1	Cup	Add to egg to make 1 1/4 cup.
Oil, Canola	1	Tablespoon	Add to egg and milk.
			Add egg & milk to dry ingredients; mix well.
			Let stand 5 min; add 1/4 cup to hot (350*) and oiled griddle. Cook until golden brown

Comments:

Serve with real maple syrup.

Serving Size 65 grams About 2.3 oz. Recipe Total Weight About 18.6 oz

Water	**Calories**	**Protein**	**Fat**	**Carbs**	**Fiber**	**Sugars**	**Phos***	**Pot***	**Sodium***
35	128	4	3	22	1	5	87	107	337

*Values are in mg. All others are in grams

Pizza, Dough; Bread Machine

Item	Quantity		Directions
			Makes about 17 ounces (473g) of dough; enough for a 16 inch Pizza.
Flour, All Purpose	2 1/8	Cup	Add to bread machine pan
Salt, table	1/2	Teaspoon	Add to pan
Sugar, White	1	Tablespoon	Add to pan
Water, tap	3/4	Cup	Add to pan
Oil, Canola	1	Tablespoon	Add to pan; Put pan in bread machine; close lid
Yeast, baker's, Dry	3/4	Teaspoon	Add to yeast cup; set machine to make pizza dough; turn on
			When done, remove form bread maker, cover with flour; knead until dough is dry. Form into pizza shell.
			Let dough rise in a 105*F oven for 90 minutes or more

Comments:

12 ounces (340g) makes a 12-inch pizza. 16 ounces (454g) makes a 16 inch pizza. Let rise in a 105*F oven until desired thickness. To heat oven to 105*F, turn on for 1 minute, then turn off.

Serving Size 468 grams About 16.5 oz. Recipe Total Weight About 16.8 oz

Water	Calories	Protein	Fat	Carbs	Fiber	Sugars	Phos*	Pot*	Sodium*
206	1,128	28	16	213	8	13	301	308	1,176

* Values are in mg. All others are in grams

Pizza, Dough; Mixer

Item	Quantity		Directions
			Makes about 1 1/2 pounds of dough; 692 grams
			Recipe for use with a mixer with a dough hook
Yeast, baker's, Dry	2	Teaspoon	Add to mixer bowl
Water, tap	1	Cup	Warm to 105 *F; add to bowl; Dissolve yeast.
Salt, table	1/2	Teaspoon	Add to bowl
Oil, Canola	2	Teaspoon	Add to bowl
Flour, All Purpose	2 1/2	Cup	Add to bowl; mix on speed 2, 1 min use dough hook.
Flour, All Purpose	1	Cup	Add flour slowly until dough cleans side of bowl.
			Knead on speed 2 for two min.
			Pizza; Roll out on counter to fit lightly oiled pizza pan or cookie sheet.

Comments:

12 ounces (340g) makes a 12 inch pizza. 16 ounces (454g) makes a 16 inch pizza.

Heat oven to 105*F; turn on for 1 minute, then turn off. Let dough rise to the desired thickness, about 20 to 30 minutes.

Serving Size 694 grams About 24.5 oz. Recipe Total Weight About 24.5 oz

Water	Calories	Protein	Fat	Carbs	Fiber	Sugars	Phos*	Pot*	Sodium*
289	1,698	48	14	337	14	1	523	544	1,202

* Values are in mg. All others are in grams

Pizza, Sausage and Onions

Item	Quantity		Directions
Pizza Dough	16	Ounce	Use 1 pound of dough for 16 inch pizza.
			Roll out to fit cookie sheet or pizza pan.
			Let rise for 15 minutes or more in an oven warmed for 1 minute.
Spaghetti sauce with meat	1	Cup	Spread evenly on rolled out dough.
Sausage, Hot Italian Homemade	8	Ounce	Cook in fry pan, crumble and spread on dough.
Onions, raw,	1/2	Cup	Slice onion 1/4 inch thick, separate rings;
			place on pizza
Mozzarella, shredded part skim	4	Ounce	Spread cheese evenly on pizza
			Bake at 450 *F for 15 - 20 minutes; cut into 8 slices

Comments:

Serving size is one slice. One slice of pizza made with commercial sausage has about 46 more grams of sodium

Serving Size 141 grams About 5 oz. Recipe Total Weight About 39.9 oz

Water	Calories	Protein	Fat	Carbs	Fiber	Sugars	Phos*	Pot*	Sodium*
85	274	13	11	31	2	4	187	285	296

* Values are in mg. All others are in grams

Pizza, Sausage, Onions, Pepperoni

Item	Quantity		Directions
			Makes 8 slices, 5 1/4 ounces (149g) each
Pizza Dough	16	Ounce	Use 1 pound of dough. Roll out to fit cookie sheet or 16 inch pizza pan.
			Warm oven for 1 minute. Let rise in oven until dough is desired thickness.
Spaghetti sauce with meat	1	Cup	Spread on dough.
Sausage, Hot Italian Homemade	8	Ounce	Cook in fry pan, crumble, spread on dough.
Onions, raw	1/2	Cup	Slice onion, chop into small pieces; place on pizza
Pepperoni, Sliced	32	Each	Place sliced pepperoni evenly on pizza.
Mozzarella, shredded, part skim	4	Ounce	Spread on dough. Bake at 450*F for 15-20 minute.

Comments:

Serving size based on eight slices. One slice of pizza made with commercial sausage has about 46 more grams of sodium.

Serving Size 149 grams About 5.3 oz. Recipe Total Weight About 42.1 oz

Water	Calories	Protein	Fat	Carbs	Fiber	Sugars	Phos*	Pot*	Sodium*
87	314	15	14	31	2	4	200	308	423

* Values are in mg. All others are in grams

Pork Barbecue Sweet

Item	Quantity		Directions
			Makes about 6 serving, 6 ounces (174g) each
Pork, Shoulder,	1 1/2	Pound	Add to crockpot
Barbeque, Sweet	1 1/2	Cup	Prepare recipe for Sweet Barbeque; Add to crockpot.
			Cook on low for 6 hours.

Comments:

Serve with egg noodles or rice.

Serving Size 174 grams   About 6.1 oz.   Recipe Total Weight   About 36.2 oz

Water	Calories	Protein	Fat	Carbs	Fiber	Sugars	Phos*	Pot*	Sodium*
126	257	21	14	10	1	8	239	584	86

* Values are in mg. All others are in grams

Pork Chops, Braised

Item	Quantity		Directions
			Makes 2, three ounce pork chops.
Oil, Canola	1	Tablespoon	Add to 10 inch fry pan, warm on medium heat
Pork Loin Chops	6	Ounce	Place 2, three ounce chops in fry pan, sear for 2 minutes on each side.
Garlic, Granulated	1/8	Teaspoon	Spread on pork chops.
Pepper, Black ground	1/8	Teaspoon	Spread on pork chops
Water, tap	1/4	Cup	Add to pan, cover, set heat to PL3. Simmer for 3 min on each side. Pour liquid into a small cup. Good on the chops.

Serving Size 120 grams About 4.2 oz. Recipe Total Weight About 8.6 oz

Water	Calories	Protein	Fat	Carbs	Fiber	Sugars	Phos*	Pot*	Sodium*
90	167	19	10	1	0	0	197	329	43

* Values are in mg. All others are in grams

Pork, General Toas

Item	Quantity		Directions
			Serves 6
Pork,	1 1/2	Pound	Cut into 1/2 x 1 inch pieces; add to crock pot
Ginger, Ground	1	Teaspoon	Add to pot
Garlic, Minced	1	Teaspoon	Add to pot
Sugar, White	1/4	Cup	Add to pot
Pepper, Red ground	1/8	Teaspoon	Add to pot
Soy Sauce, low sodium	1/2	Tablespoon	Add to pot
Vinegar, Cider	1/2	Cup	Add to pot
Wine, table red	1/2	Cup	Add to pot
			Cook in crock pot on low for 4 hours;

Comments:

Serve with rice or egg noodles.

Serving Size 120 grams About 4.2 oz. Recipe Total Weight About 34.6 oz

Water	Calories	Protein	Fat	Carbs	Fiber	Sugars	Phos*	Pot*	Sodium*
85	197	15	10	7	0	6	166	305	86

* Values are in mg. All others are in grams

Pork, Mammoth Barbecue

Item	Quantity		Directions
			Makes 8 servings, 4 ounces (114g) each
Pork, Shoulder,	1 1/2	Pound	Add to crockpot
Barbecue Sauce, Mammoth	1 1/2	Cup	Add to crockpot
			Cook on low for 6 hours

Comments:

Serve over egg noodles or rice.

Serving Size 120 grams About 4.2 oz. Recipe Total Weight About 37 oz

Water	Calories	Protein	Fat	Carbs	Fiber	Sugars	Phos*	Pot*	Sodium*
86	181	14	10	8	1	7	167	449	58

* Values are in mg. All others are in grams

Pork, General Toas Stir Fry

Item	Quantity		Directions
			Makes about 4 servings,
			Prepare the recipe for Gen Toas Sauce; set aside.
Pork, Shoulder,	1	Pound	Slice pork 1/4 thick; then cut into 1 inch squares; set aside.
Onion; medium;	1	Each	Slice onion 1/4 inch thick; cut in half; set aside.
Peppers, Bell	1/2	Cup	Slice half a pepper into 1/4 inch strips; cut in half; set aside.
Celery,	1	Cup	Chop celery into 1/4 inch slices, then cut in half; set aside.
Vegetables, frozen,	5	Ounce	Thaw 1/2 package of broccoli or oriental veggies; set aside.
Oil, Canola	2	Tablespoon	Add to large (12inch) pry pan; Place on medium heat.
			Add pork to pan; sauté on medium heat until cooked.
Gen Toas Sauce	1	Cup	Add Gen Toas Sauce to fry pan.
			Add onions, peppers, celery and veggies to fry pan; sauté for 5 minutes until veggies are tender.
			Add water if needed.

Comments:

Serve over rice.

Serving Size 227 grams About 8 oz. Recipe Total Weight About 38.7 oz.

Water	Calories	Protein	Fat	Carbs	Fiber	Sugars	Phos*	Pot*	Sodium*
174	297	18	18	15	2	7	216	491	263

*Values are in mg. All others are in grams

Pork Pot Roast with Gravy

Item	Quantity		Directions
			Serves 4
Pork, Shoulder,	2	Pound	Add to large fry pan with a tight lid
Pepper, Black ground	1/2	Teaspoon	Add to fry pan
Garlic, Granulated	1/2	Teaspoon	Add to pan
Sage, dry ground	1	Teaspoon	Add to fry pan
Marjoram, dried	2	Teaspoon	Add to pan
Water, tap	1	Cup	Add to fry pan; bring to boil; simmer 2 hrs. Add water as necessary; bottom of pan should always be covered.
			Remove pork from pan; place on a platter; Pour liquid from pot roast pan into 4 cup Pyrex measuring cup.
Water, tap	1	Cup	Add water to make 2 cups; stir and return to fry pan on low heat.
Flour, All Purpose	4	Tablespoon	Add flour to a pint shaker jar with lid.
Water, tap	1	Cup	Add water to shaker jar, put on lid, shake until all flour is mixed. Wisk flour into fry pan; whisk until smooth; cook on medium heat.
			Stir constantly until thick; add water if necessary; simmer 2 min. Add flour water mixture if too thin.

Comments:

4 tablespoons of gravy is about 60 grams or 2 ounces; a dash of salt = 155 milligrams of sodium; 1/8 teaspoon of salt is about 307 milligrams of sodium. Be careful if you add salt.

Serving Size 240 grams About 8.5 oz. Recipe Total Weight About 58.3 oz

Water	Calories	Protein	Fat	Carbs	Fiber	Sugars	Phos*	Pot*	Sodium*
195	263	24	16	4	0	0	257	433	85

* Values are in mg. All others are in grams

Potato Casserole

Item	Quantity		Directions
			Makes 10 servings, 6 ounces (170g) each.
Potato, Raw.	6	Cup	Peel, Slice thin; add to 8 cup bowl.
Sausage, Hot Italian Homemade	8	Ounce	Crumble and add to large fry pan.
Beef, Ground 80%; raw	3/4	Pound	Add 12 ounces to frypan, crumble, cook; set aside.
Butter	3	Tablespoon	Add to large casserole bowl with lid.
Pepper, Black ground	1	Teaspoon	Add to bowl
Garlic, Granulated	1	Teaspoon	Add to bowl and mix.
			Add meat, cover. Microwave on Hi for 20 min or until potatoes are cooked.
Mozzarella, shredded, part skim	8	Ounce	Add to bowl and mix.
			Microwave on Hi to melt cheese.

Comments:

This recipe is high in potassium at 580 milligrams for 1 serving of 6 ounces. An 8 ounce serving contains 775 milligrams. It is one of my favorite meals.

Serving Size 170 grams…..About 6 oz. Recipe Total Weight About 61.5 oz

Water	Calories	Protein	Fat	Carbs	Fiber	Sugars	Phos*	Pot*	Sodium*
115	301	17	18	17	2	1	267	582	236

* Values are in mg. All others are in grams

Potatoes, Fried

Item	Quantity		Directions
Potato,	8	Ounce	Cut 2 small potatoes into 1/8 inch thick slices. Place on a microwaveable dish. Microwave on Hi for 4 min; set aside
Oil, Canola	2	Tablespoon	Add to large fry pan; set heat to medium
			Add potatoes to fry pan; spread out; fry on 1 side until brown.
Onion	1/3	Cup	Dice raw onion to fill 1/3 cup.
			Flip potatoes and add onions.
			Fry on medium heat until onions soft: serve hot.
			Makes 2 servings about 4 1/2 ounces (127g) each

Comments:

This recipe is high in potassium at 431 mg per 4.5 ounce serving.

Serving Siz) 127 grams…..About 4.5 oz. Recipe Total Weight About 10.8 oz.

Water	Calories	Protein	Fat	Carbs	Fiber	Sugars	Phos*	Pot*	Sodium*
94	180	2	11	19	2	2	60	431	7

* Values are in mg. All others are in grams

Potatoes, Whipped

Item	Quantity		Directions
			Makes about 5 servings of 4 ounces (112g) each
Potatoes, white	1	Pound	Wash 4 small potatoes; peel; slice 1/2 thick; place in 4qt pot.
			Cover potatoes with water boil until soft; drain.
Butter	2	Tablespoon	Cut butter into 1/8 inch pats; add to pan.
Cream, heavy whipping	1/4	Cup	Add to pan
Pepper, Black ground	1/4	Teaspoon	Add to pan
Garlic, Granulated	1/2	Teaspoon	Add to pan; whip with hand mixer until smooth; serve.

Serving Size 112 grams About 4 oz. Recipe Total Weight About 19.2 oz

Water	Calories	Protein	Fat	Carbs	Fiber	Sugars	Phos*	Pot*	Sodium*
80	166	2	9	19	2	1	48	325	46

* Values are in mg. All others are in grams

Red Cabbage, cooked

Item	Quantity		Directions
			Makes a big pot full; about 9 servings, 4 ounces (120g) each
Cabbage, Red,	8	Cup	Add 8 cups of shredded cabbage to 8 cup Pyrex measuring dish
Sugar, Brown	1/2	Cup	Add to dish
Vinegar, Cider	1/2	Cup	Add to dish
Water, tap	1	Cup	Add to dish
Bacon, slice	4	Each	Chop 4 slices into small pieces; add to dish.
			Cook on power level 10 in micro wave for 40 min or until tender. Stir every 10 min.
			Check liquid in pot every 10 minutes; don't let the pot get dry.

Serving Size 120 grams About 4.2 oz. Recipe Total Weight About 38.8 oz

Water	Calories	Protein	Fat	Carbs	Fiber	Sugars	Phos*	Pot*	Sodium*
99	100	3	5	12	1	10	40	193	112

* Values are in mg. All others are in grams

Rice

Item	Quantity		Directions
			Do not salt the water when cooking rice.
			Makes about 3.5 servings of 1 cup each which is
			about 5.6 ounces (158g) each.
Rice, White, long grain	1	Cup	Add to 2 quart pot with lid.
Water, tap	2	Cup	Add to pot; bring to low boil. Put on lid and cook on low for 14 minutes.
			Let stand 10 min; rinse if desired.

Comments:

Makes about 3 1/2 cups; ---1 cup of rice is about 158g or 5.6 ounces.

Serving Size 158 grams About 5.6 oz. Recipe Total Weight About 19.6 oz

Water	Calories	Protein	Fat	Carbs	Fiber	Sugars	Phos*	Pot*	Sodium*
108	206	4	0	45	1	0	68	55	2

* Values are in mg. All others are in grams

Sausage, Breakfast, High salt

Item	Quantity		Directions
			Makes 1 pound of sausage.
Pork, Ground shoulder	1	Pound	Add ground pork to a medium size bowl; flatten out.
Sausage seasoning, Breakfast Homemade; HI salt	4	Teaspoon	Sprinkle 2 teaspoons of seasoning on meat.
			Fold over and press down.
			Sprinkle 2 more teaspoons of seasoning on meat.
			Fold over and press down.
			Mix well using a big spoon.
			Keep folding over and mixing until evenly mixed.

Comments:

Salty like store bought breakfast sausage. Make 1 ounce patties, press thin and fry. Makes a good egg and sausage sandwich.

Serving Size 30 grams About 1.1 oz. Recipe Total Weight About 16.3 oz.

Water	Calories	Protein	Fat	Carbs	Fiber	Sugars	Phos*	Pot*	Sodium*
19	70	5	5	0	0	0	54	92	157

* Values are in mg. All others are in grams

Sausage, Breakfast, Low Salt

Item	Quantity		Directions
			Makes 1 pound of sausage
Pork, Ground shoulder	1	Pound	Add ground pork to a medium size bowl; flatten out.
Sausage seasoning, Breakfast Homemade; LOW salt	4	Teaspoon	Sprinkle 2 teaspoons of seasoning on meat. Fold over and press down.
			Sprinkle 2 more teaspoons of seasoning on meat. Fold over and press down.
			Mix well using a big spoon. Keep folding over and mixing until evenly mixed.

Comments:

Much lower salt than store bought breakfast sausage ---Make 1 ounce patties and press thin;--Makes a good egg and sausage sandwich.

Serving Size 30 grams About 1.1 oz. Recipe Total Weight About 16.2 oz.

Water	Calories	Protein	Fat	Carbs	Fiber	Sugars	Phos*	Pot*	Sodium*
19	71	5	5	0	0	0	54	93	73

* Values are in mg. All others are in grams

Sausage, Breakfast, Medium salt

Item	Quantity		Directions
			Makes 1 pound of sausage
Pork, Ground shoulder	1	Pound	Add ground pork to a medium size bowl; flatten out
Sausage seasoning, Breakfast Homemade; Medium salt	4	Teaspoon	Sprinkle 2 teaspoons of seasoning on meat. Fold over and press down.
			Sprinkle 2 more teaspoons of seasoning on meat. Fold over and press down.
			Mix well using a big spoon. Keep folding over and mixing until evenly mixed.

Comments:

Less salty than store bought breakfast sausage. One ounce makes a thin, 3-inch patty just right for an egg sandwich or muffin.

Serving Size 30 grams About 1.1 oz. Recipe Total Weight About 16.3 oz.

Water	Calories	Protein	Fat	Carbs	Fiber	Sugars	Phos*	Pot*	Sodium*
19	70	5	5	0	0	0	54	92	117

* Values are in mg. All others are in grams

Sausage, Hot Italian

Item	Quantity		Directions
			Makes about 8 servings, 4 ounces (113g) each.
Pork, shoulder Ground	2	Pound	Add ground pork to medium bowl; flatten out.
Italian Sausage Seasoning	1 1/2	Tablespoon	Spread ½ tablespoon evenly on pork. Fold over and mix. Repeat until all seasoning is used and is evenly mixed.

Comments:

Yummy --- a big Kitchen Aid mixer is really handy for doing this.

Serving Size 113 grams About 4 oz. Recipe Total Weight About 32.4 oz

Water	Calories	Protein	Fat	Carbs	Fiber	Sugars	Phos*	Pot*	Sodium*
72	267	19	20	1	0	0	207	354	174

* Values are in mg. All others are in grams

Scrapple, with pork only

Item	Quantity		Directions
			Makes 2 loaf pans 8.5x4.5x2.5
Pork, Shoulder,	2	Pound	Cut to 1 inch thick strips, add to 4 qt pot
Water, tap	4	Cup	Add water to pot to cover meat
Sage, dry ground	1	Tablespoon	Add to pot
Pepper, Black ground	2	Teaspoon	Add to pot
Salt, table	1/2	Teaspoon	Add to pot
Thyme, dried Leaves	2	Teaspoon	Add to pot
Savory, ground	2	Teaspoon	Add to pot
			Simmer Pork until shredable; about 2 hrs.
			Pour stock into 8 cup measure cup.
Water, tap	2	Cup	Add water to stock to make 4 cups. Shred the pork, return it to the pot and bring it to a boil.
Cornmeal; yellow	2	Cup	Place in 4 cup measuring cup.
Water, tap	1 1/2	Cup	Add to corn meal and stir until all the cornmeal is wet.
			Remove stock from heat; Slowly add corn meal to the pot; Stir constantly. Cook mixture on low heat until very thick; at least 3 minutes. Stir constantly.
			Press tightly into 2 loaf pans; cool in refrigerator until set.
			Cut into 3/8 inch slices. Fry over med heat until crisp.

Comments:

Good with eggs and toast, ---made with pork only, no scraps or organ meat.

Serving Size 120 grams About 4.2 oz. Recipe Total Weight About 103.8 oz

Water	Calories	Protein	Fat	Carbs	Fiber	Sugars	Phos*	Pot*	Sodium*
99	106	7	5	8	1	0	95	152	77

*Values are in mg. All others are in grams

Spaghetti Sauce with Meat

Item	Quantity		Directions
			Makes about 3.5 quarts; shows 1/2 cup serving
Tomato Puree, 28oz can, no salt	3	Can	Add to large crock pot
Water, tap	1	Cup	Add 1/2 can to pot
Oregano	1	Tablespoon	Add to pot
Basil, dried leaves	1	Tablespoon	Add to pot
Parsley, dried	1	Tablespoon	Add to pot
Garlic, Minced	1	Tablespoon	Add to pot
Sugar, White	2	Tablespoon	Add to pot
Beef, Ground 80%; raw	8	Ounce	Crumble and add to pot
Sausage, Hot Italian Homemade	8	Ounce	Crumble and add to pot
Pepper, Red ground	1/8	Teaspoon	Add to pot: Cook in microwave on Hi until bubbling;
			About 25 min. Cook in crock pot on Hi for 4 hours.

Comments:

Very high in potassium; so, use sparingly.

Serving Size(g) 120 grams About 4.2 oz. Recipe Total Weight About 112.9 oz.

Water	Calories	Protein	Fat	Carbs	Fiber	Sugars	Phos*	Pot*	Sodium*
101	83	5	3	10	2	5	68	466	46

* Values are in mg. All others are in grams

Soup Chicken and Broth

Item	Quantity		Directions
			Makes2 servings, about 1 cup each.
Chicken Broth, low sodium	1	Cup	Add to 2 qt pot
Pepper, Black ground	1/4	Teaspoon	Add to pot
Poultry Seasoning, Homemade		Teaspoon	Add to pot
Garlic, Granulated	1/8	Teaspoon	Add to pot
Celery Seed	1/8	Teaspoon	Add to pot
Chicken, Breast, no skin or bone	6	Ounce	Slice into strips ¼ inch by 1 inch. Add to pot.
			Simmer until chicken is cooked.
			Serve with elbows or other small pasta.

Serving Size 205 grams   About 7.2 oz.   Recipe Total Weight   About 14.5 oz

Water	Calories	Protein	Fat	Carbs	Fiber	Sugars	Phos*	Pot*	Sodium*
181	102	19	3	1	0	0	192	393	424

* Values are in mg. All others are in grams

Soup Lentil

Item	Quantity		Directions
			Makes about 6 servings; 8 ounces (227g) each.
Lentils, Dry	1/2	Pound	Add to 4 Quart pot.
Water, tap	4	Cup	Add to 4 Quart pot.
Ham, cured,	1/2	Cup	Dice, Add to pot.
Sausage, Hot Italian Homemade	1/4	Pound	Crumble and add to pot.
Marjoram, dried	1/2	Teaspoon	Add to pot.
Oregano	1/4	Teaspoon	Add to pot.
Pepper, Black ground	1/2	Teaspoon	Add to pot.
Onions	1/2	Cup	Dice onion, add to pot.
			Bring to boil then simmer on low heat until lentils are soft; about 20 minutes.

Serving Size 227 grams About 8 oz. Recipe Total Weight About 50.8 oz.

Water	Calories	Protein	Fat	Carbs	Fiber	Sugars	Phos*	Pot*	Sodium*
182	192	14	5	24	4	1	164	354	177

* Values are in mg. All others are in grams

Pancakes; Sour Dough Starter

Item	Quantity		Directions
Flour, All Purpose	1	Cup	Add to glass bowl.
Sugar, White	1/2	Cup	Add to bowl; Set aside.
Water, tap	1	Cup	Warm in small bowl to 105*F.
Yeast, baker's, Dry	2 1/2	Teaspoon	Add yeast to water and dissolve.
			Add water and yeast to dry ingredients; mix well. Cover
			Bowl. Let stand at room temperature for 48 hrs.
			Remove from fridge and bring to 105*F before using.
			Replace used portion with equal amount of flour and water.

Serving Size 116 grams About 4.1 oz. Recipe Total Weight About 16.7 oz

Water	Calories	Protein	Fat	Carbs	Fiber	Sugars	Phos*	Pot*	Sodium*
62	215	4	1	49	1	25	49	57	5

* Values are in mg. All others are in grams

Stuffing

Item	Quantity		Directions
Butter	8	Tablespoon	Place in large frypan.
Poultry Seasoning, Homemade	1	Tablespoon	Add to pan.
Onions	1	Cup	Chop medium onion; add to pan.
Mushrooms, white, raw	1 1/2	Cup	Chopped; add to pan.
Celery, raw, cup chopped	1 1/2	Cup	Chopped; add to pan.
Sausage, Hot Italian Homemade	1/2	Pound	Break up and add to pan.
			Sauté till sausage is cooked.
Bread, white slice, store	20	Each	Cube a 1 lb loaf, add to large bowl.
			Add pan contents to bowl, mix well.

Serving Size 60 grams About 2.1 oz. Recipe Total Weight About 48 oz.

Water	Calories	Protein	Fat	Carbs	Fiber	Sugars	Phos*	Pot*	Sodium*
34	135	4	7	14	1	2	53	111	183

* Values are in mg. All others are in grams

Sweet Potato, candied

Item	Quantity		Directions
			Makes 23 ounces (652g). Sserving size is about 2 ounces.
Sweet Potato	20	Ounce	Wash 3 medium sweet potatoes; slice 1/2 inch thick.
			Place flat in a 7x11 glass pan.
Sugar, Brown	6	Tablespoon	Spread on top of sweet potatoes.
Cinnamon, Ground	1/2	Teaspoon	Sprinkle on top of sweet potatoes.
Nutmeg	1/8	Teaspoon	Sprinkle on top of sweet potatoes.
Butter	2	Tablespoon	Cut into 1/8 pats and place evenly on sweet potatoes.
			Cook in microwave, on power level 5, for 15 min or
			bake in oven for 30 min at 350 *F.

Serving Size 60 grams About 2.1 oz. Recipe Total Weight About 23 oz

Water	Calories	Protein	Fat	Carbs	Fiber	Sugars	Phos*	Pot*	Sodium*
41	83	1	2	16	2	7	26	184	47

* Values are in mg. All others are in grams

Taco Meat

Item	Quantity		Directions
			Makes about 6 servings, 4 ounces (115g) each.
Beef, Ground 80%	1	Pound	Add to large fry pan; cook and remove melted fat.
Garlic, Granulated	1	Teaspoon	Add to pan.
Ketchup	3/4	Cup	Add cup to pan.
Hot Sauce, Franks	2	Tablespoon	Add to pan.
Pepper, Red ground	1/4	Teaspoon	Add to pan.
Chili Powder, Homemade	1	Teaspoon	Add to pan; simmer for 5 minutes. Serve

Comments:

Sue's easy, quick recipe for making tacos

Serving Size 115grams About 4.1 oz. Recipe Total Weight About 24.5 oz.

Water	Calories	Protein	Fat	Carbs	Fiber	Sugars	Phos*	Pot*	Sodium*
75	229	13	15	10	0	7	132	340	359

* Values are in mg. All others are in grams

Teriyaki Beef and Peppers

Item	Quantity		Directions
			Makes 4, six-ounce (182 gm) servings.
Teriyaki Sauce	1	Each	Make Teriyaki Sauce; set aside
Oil, Canola	1	Tablespoon	Add to fry pan.
Beef, steak	1	Pound	Cut beef into ¼ inch slices; add to frypan; sauté on medium heat.
Peppers, Bell	1	Cup	Add to fry pan.
Onion; medium	1	Each	Add to fry pan; sauté until peppers are tender.
			Add Teriyaki sauce to frypan; simmer 5 minutes.
			Serve over rice.

Serving Size 182 grams About 6.4 oz. Recipe Total Weight About 36.6 oz

Water	Calories	Protein	Fat	Carbs	Fiber	Sugars	Phos*	Pot*	Sodium*
137	243	17	13	13	1	10	164	335	214

* Values are in mg. All others are in grams

Tuna, Creamed

Item	Quantity		Directions
			Makes about 8 servings; 4 ounces (115g) each.
Butter	3	Tablespoon	Add to 1 quart pyrex dish; melt in micro wave.
Flour, All Purpose	3	Tablespoon	Add to 1qt bowl.
Salt, table	1/8	Teaspoon	Add to 1qt bowl; mix with whisk until smooth.
Milk; skim	1 1/2	Cup	Slowly add to bowl while whisking briskly; mix well
			Microwave on high, stirring every minute until thick
Tunafish in water (5 oz can)	2	Can	Flake and add to 1qt bowl.
Poultry Seasoning, Homemade	1/2	Teaspoon	Add to 1quartt bowl.
Pepper, Black ground	1/8	Teaspoon	Add to 1quart bowl.
Peas, Frozen	1/2	Cup	Add to 1quart bowl.
Corn, frozen	1/2	Cup	Add to 1quart bowl; mix well.
			Cook in microwave for 5 minutes on high stirring every minute.
			Serve on toast or baking powder biscuits.

Serving Size 115 grams About 4.1 oz. Recipe Total Weight About 30.2 oz

Water	Calories	Protein	Fat	Carbs	Fiber	Sugars	Phos*	Pot*	Sodium*
90	120	10	5	9	1	3	124	192	202

* Values are in mg. All others are in grams

Tuna and Noodles

Item	Quantity		Directions
			Makes 10 servings; 4 ounces (115g) each
Egg noodles	8	Ounce	Boil in 8cup pot for 10 minutes; drain and set aside.
Tunafish in water (5 oz can)	3	Can	Add to large glass dish.
Soup, Cream of Mushroom	1	Can	Add to large glass dish.
Pepper, Black ground	1	Teaspoon	Add to glass dish.
Milk; skim	1/2	Cup	Add to large glass dish.
			Add cooked noodles to glass dish, mix.
American Cheese, Slice	6	Each	Layer cheese in middle and on top of noodles.
			Cook in microwave on power level 7 until cheese is melted. Stir every minute after cheese starts to melt.

Comments:

This is not a kidney friendly recipe; --There is too much salt-- so be careful how much you eat.

Serving Size 115 grams **About 4.1 oz.** **Recipe Total Weight** **About 44 oz**

Water	Calories	Protein	Fat	Carbs	Fiber	Sugars	Phos*	Pot*	Sodium*
85	146	12	7	9	0	1	187	138	556

* Values are in mg. All others are in grams

Tuna Salad

Item	Quantity		Directions
			Makes 8.1 ounces (230g); enough for 2 small sandwiches, or 1 large sandwich.
Tunafish in water (5 oz can)	1	Can	Place in small bowl.
Miracle Whip	2	Tablespoon	Add to bowl.
Onion	2	Tablespoon	Dice and add to bowl.
Pickle, Bread and Butter	5	Each	Dice 5 slices and add to bowl; mix.
Pepper, Black ground	1/8	Teaspoon	Add to bowl, mix.

Comments:

Serving size is 115 grams; enough for 1 sandwich. High in soudium

Serving Size 115 grams **About 4.1 oz.** **Recipe Total Weight** **About 8.1 oz**

Water	Calories	Protein	Fat	Carbs	Fiber	Sugars	Phos*	Pot*	Sodium*
79	123	14	4	7	0	5	121	283	363

* Values are in mg. All others are in grams

Waffles, Belgian

Item	Quantity		Directions
			Makes 4 waffles, 8.2 ounces (234g) each.
Flour, All Purpose	1 3/4	Cup	Add to 8 cup mixing bowl.
Cornstarch	4	Tablespoon	Add to bowl.
Sugar, White	2	Tablespoon	Add to bowl.
Baking Powder	3	Teaspoon	Add to bowl.
Cinnamon, Ground	1	Teaspoon	Add to bowl.
Salt, table	1/8	Teaspoon	Add to bowl.
Milk; skim	1 3/4	Cup	Add to bowl slowly and stir until all flour is wet.
Eggs, large	2	Each	Add to bowl and mix well.
Oil, Canola	1/2	Cup	Add to bowl.
Vanilla extract	1	Teaspoon	Add to bowl and mix.
			Add 1/2 cup batter to hot waffle iron; cook till crisp; 3-4 min

Comments:

1/4 waffle is 58.5g (about 2 ounces).

Serving Size 234 grams About 8.3 oz. Recipe Total Weight About 33 oz

Water	Calories	Protein	Fat	Carbs	Fiber	Sugars	Phos*	Pot*	Sodium*
125	574	12	30	63	2	12	294	266	523

* Values are in mg. All others are in grams

Salads

Tossed salad, no dressing

Item	Quantity		Directions
			Small individual side salad; no dressing.
Lettuce, iceberg	28	Gram	Cut into bite size pieces; add to small salad bowl
Apples, 3" peeled	15	Gram	Slice apple into 1/4 inch thick slices; chop, add to bowl.
Cheese, Cheddar, brick	15	Gram	Slice cheese 1/8 inch thick; cut into smaller pieces; add to bowl.
Pepperoni, Sliced	2	Each	Cut 2 slices into 4 pieces each; add to bowl.
Cucumber, peeled	20	Gram	Slice 1/4 inch thick; cut into quarters; add to bowl.
Onions, thin slice	10	Gram	Cut 1 slice into smaller pieces; add to bowl

Comments:

Good with French, sweet Italian or other dressing.

Serving Size 93 grams About 3.3 oz. Recipe Total Weight About 3.2 oz

Water	Calories	Protein	Fat	Carbs	Fiber	Sugars	Phos*	Pot*	Sodium*
76	99	5	7	5	1	3	92	122	169

* Values are in mg. All others are in grams

Tossed salad, French Dressing

Item	Quantity		Directions
			Small individual salad with French dressing.
Lettuce, iceberg	20	Gram	Shred; add to salad bowl.
Cheese, Cheddar, brick	15	Gram	Add to bowl.
Pepperoni, Sliced	2	Each	Cut 2 slices into 4 pieces each; add to bowl.
Cucumber, peeled	28	Gram	Cut 4 slices 1/8 inch thick; cut slices in half; add to bowl.
Dressing, French	1	Tablespoon	Spread on salad.

Comments:

Also good with Italian or Russian dressing.

Serving Size 82 grams About 2.9 oz. Recipe Total Weight About 2.9 oz.

Water	Calories	Protein	Fat	Carbs	Fiber	Sugars	Phos*	Pot*	Sodium*
58	160	5	15	3	1	2	87	105	210

* Values are in mg. All others are in grams

Tossed Salad, Italian Dressing

Item	Quantity		Directions
			Small side salad with Italian dressing.
Lettuce, iceberg	20	Gram	Shred and add to bowl.
Cheese, Cheddar, brick	15	Gram	Add to bowl.
Pepperoni, Sliced	2	Each	Cut 2 slices into 4 pieces each and add to bowl.
Cucumber, peeled	28	Gram	Cut 4 slices 1/8 inch thick, cut in half, add to bowl.
Dressing, Italian	1	Tablespoon	Spread on salad.

Comments:

Also good with French dressing.

Serving Size 80 grams About 2.8 oz. Recipe Total Weight About 2.8 oz.

Water	Calories	Protein	Fat	Carbs	Fiber	Sugars	Phos*	Pot*	Sodium*
56	171	5	16	2	1	1	85	95	218

* Values are in mg. All others are in grams

Cheese, Cucumber, Pepperoni French

Item	Quantity		Directions
			Small individual salad. No dressing.
Lettuce, iceberg	20	Gram	Shred; add to salad bowl.
Cheese, Cheddar, brick	15	Gram	Add to bowl.
Pepperoni, Sliced	2	Each	Cut 2 slices into 4 pieces each; add to bowl.
Cucumber, peeled	20	Gram	Cut 4 slices 1/8 inch thick; cut slices in half; add to bowl
Dressing, French	1	Tablespoon	Spread on salad.

Comments:

Also good with Italian or Russian dressing.

Serving Size 74 grams About 2.6 oz. Recipe Total Weight About 2.6 oz.

Water	Calories	Protein	Fat	Carbs	Fiber	Sugars	Phos*	Pot*	Sodium*
51	159	5	15	3	0	2	85	94	210

* Values are in mg. All others are in grams

Lettuce and Onion salad

Item	Quantity		Directions
Lettuce, iceberg	1	Ounce	Cut into bite size pieces; add to small salad bowl,
Onions, raw, slice, thin	1/2	Ounce	Cut into bite size pieces; add to small salad bowl,

Comments:

Good with French, sweet Italian or most other salad dressings.

Serving Size 43 About 1.5 oz. Recipe Total Weight About 1.5 oz

Water	Calories	Protein	Fat	Carbs	Fiber	Sugars	Phos*	Pot*	Sodium*
40	10	1	0	2	1	1	12	64	4

* Values are in mg. All others are in grams

Macaroni Salad with Onion and Pickle

Item	Quantity		Directions
			Makes 7 cups.
Elbows	1.5	Cups	fill 4 qt sauce pan half full with water; bring to boil
			Add DRY elbows and 2 large eggs to a 4 quart pot. Boil for ten minutes. Drain. Add elbows to large mixing bowl.
			Cool eggs in ice water, Set aside.
Tuna fish in water (5 oz can)	2	Can	Drain; Shred and add to bowl.
Mayonnaise, regular	2	Tablespoon	Add to bowl.
Miracle Whip	2	Tablespoon	Add to bowl.
Eggs, large	2	Each	Dice hard boiled eggs and Add to bowl.
Onions	1	Cup	Dice 1/2 medium onion; add to bowl.
Pickle, Bread & Butter	10	Each	Dice ten pickle slices and add to bowl. Mix well.

Comments:

1 cup of Macaroni salad weighs 5.3 oz 150 grams 1 cup dry elbows boiled for 10 minutes yields 2 3/4 cups of cooked elbows

Serving Size 150 grams   About 5.3 oz.   Recipe Total Weight   About 40.8 oz.

Water	Calories	Protein	Fat	Carbs	Fiber	Sugars	Phos*	Pot*	Sodium*
104	200	13	6	24	2	3	125	183	204

* Values are in mg. All others are in grams

Macaroni Salad with Tuna

Item	Quantity		Directions
			Makes about 3 cups. 4 small servings.
Elbows	1	Cup	Boil for 10 min; drain; add to mixing bowl.
Mayonnaise, regular	1/2	Cup	Add to bowl.
Onions	1/2	Cup	Diced onion, Add to bowl.
Peppers, Bell,	1/4	Cup	Dice peppers, Add to bowl.
Tuna fish in water (5 oz can)	1	Can	Add to bowl.
Vinegar, Cider	1/2	Teaspoon	Add to bowl, mix well.

Serving Size 120 grams About 4.2 oz. Recipe Total Weight About 17.3 oz.

Water	Calories	Protein	Fat	Carbs	Fiber	Sugars	Phos*	Pot*	Sodium*
78	268	9	21	11	1	1	78	125	257

* Values are in mg. All others are in grams

Pasta Salad, Bow Tie

Item	Quantity		Directions
			Makes about 4 servings, 4 ounces (120 grams) each
Pasta, bow ties dry	1	Cup	Boil for 10 minutes in 2 quart pot. Drain, add to bowl.
Celery	1/4	Cup	Cut celery into ¼ inch slices, chop. Add to bowl.
Peppers, Bell,	2	Tablespoon	Chop into ½ inch pieces. Add to bowl.
Carrots	2	Tablespoon	Add Finely Chopped carrots to bowl'
Onions	2	Tablespoon	Dice and add to bowl. Set aside.
Pepper, Black ground	1/8	Teaspoon	Add to a small bowl.
Mayonnaise, regular	2/3	Cup	Add to bowl.
Sugar, White	1/2	Teaspoon	Add to bowl.
Lemon Juice	1	Tablespoon	Add to bowl, mix and add to pasta. Mix well and chill.

Serving Size 120 grams About 4.2 oz. Recipe Total Weight About 18.4 oz.

Water	Calories	Protein	Fat	Carbs	Fiber	Sugars	Phos*	Pot*	Sodium*
67	338	4	26	22	2	2	50	80	223

* Values are in mg. All others are in grams

Tuna Salad

Item	Quantity		Directions
			Makes 7.5 ounces (212g); enough for 2 small sandwiches, or 1 large sandwich.
Tuna fish in water (5 oz can)	1	Can	Shred tuna and place in small bowl.
Miracle Whip	2	Tablespoon	Add to bowl.
Onions	2	Tablespoon	Dice; add to bowl.
Pickle, Bread & Butter;	5	Each	Dice 5 slices; add to bowl; mix.
Pepper, Black ground	1/8	Teaspoon	Add to bowl, mix.

Comments:

Serving size is one half of recipe or about 115 grams; enough for 1 sandwich.

Serving Size 115 grams About 4.1 oz. Recipe Total Weight About 8.1 oz.

Water	Calories	Protein	Fat	Carbs	Fiber	Sugars	Phos*	Pot*	Sodium*
79	123	14	4	7	0	5	121	283	363

* Values are in mg. All others are in grams

Sandwiches:

Beef, Shaved Steak

Item	Quantity		Directions
			Makes 2 large sandwiches
Mushrooms, white,	1	Cup	Slice 4 medium mushrooms about 1/4 inch thick; add to 2 cup measure
Onions	1/2	Cup	Cut 1/4 inch slices from an onion; chop; add to cup.
Peppers, sweet, green	1/4	Cup	Chop about 1 quarter of a pepper, add to cup.
			Cover cup, microwave on hi for 2 minutes; set aside
Oil, Canola	1	Tablespoon	Add to large fry pan.
Beef, shaved steak	3	Ounce	Add shaved steak to fry pan.
Thyme, dried Leaves	1/2	Teaspoon	Add to fry pan.
Garlic, Granulated	1/2	Teaspoon	Add to fry pan.
Marjoram, dried	1/2	Teaspoon	Add to fry pan.
Pepper, Black ground	1/8	Teaspoon	Add to fry pan.
Salt, table	1/8	Teaspoon	Add to fry pan, simmer until beef is done.
			Add veggies and simmer for 1 minute.
Rolls Italian	8	Ounce	Use 2 rolls made from pizza dough, 4 oz each
			Spread half of mixture on each roll.
Mozzarella, shredded	1/2	Cup	Spread 1/4 cup cheese on each roll; broil until cheese melts. Enjoy

Serving Size 60 grams About 2.1 oz. Recipe Total Weight About 20.2 oz

Water	Calories	Protein	Fat	Carbs	Fiber	Sugars	Phos*	Pot*	Sodium*
37	112	5	5	13	1	1	75	101	136

* Values are in mg. All others are in grams

Hotdog and Roll

Item	Quantity		Directions
			Serves 1
Hot Dogs, beef & pork	1	Each	Microwave for 1 min; fry with a little oil until brown.
Rolls, Hotdog	1	Each	Combine hotdog and roll.
Mustard, yellow	1	Teaspoon	Spread on roll.

Serving Size 92 grams About 3.2 oz. Recipe Total Weight About 3.2 oz

Water	Calories	Protein	Fat	Carbs	Fiber	Sugars	Phos*	Pot*	Sodium*
44	257	10	14	22	1	4	88	136	634

* Values are in mg. All others are in grams

Peanut Butter and Jelly Sandwich

Item	Quantity		Directions
			Makes 1 serving
Bread, white slice, store	2	Each	Spread with peanut butter.
Peanut Butter	2	Tablespoon	Spread evenly on bread.
Jelly, Strawberry	1 1/2	Tablespoon	Spread evenly on bread.

Serving Size 124 grams About 4.4 oz. Recipe Total Weight About 4.4 oz

Water	Calories	Protein	Fat	Carbs	Fiber	Sugars	Phos*	Pot*	Sodium*
32	435	13	19	59	4	23	169	273	447

* Values are in mg. All others are in grams

Red Ruben

Item	Quantity		Directions
			Recipe is for 1 open face Rubin Sandwich
			Make Russian dressing ahead of time; set aside
			Warm 3 ounces (90 gm) of corned beef for each sandwich; set aside.
			Warm 1/2 cup red cabbage in micro wave for each sandwich set aside.
Bread, Pumpernickel,	1	Each	About 1oz slice.
Butter, salted, pat (	1	Each	Spread small amount of butter on one side of bread.
			Fry bread in a large fry pan until bottom is toasted.
Corned Beef	3	Ounce	Arrange evenly on toasted bread.
Dressing, Russian	2	Tablespoon	Arrange evenly on corned beef.
Red Cabbage, Cooked	1/2	Cup	Arrange evenly on sandwich.
Cheese, Swiss slice	2	Each	Place Swiss cheese on top of cabbage.
			Place sandwich in broiler until cheese is melted.
			Serve while hot.

Comments:

Serve with extra Russian dressing.

Serving Size 240 grams About 8.5 oz. Recipe Total Weight About 8.5 oz.

Water	Calories	Protein	Fat	Carbs	Fiber	Sugars	Phos*	Pot*	Sodium*
131	570	30	38	27	2	10	414	464	1,397

* Values are in mg. All others are in grams

Roast Beef, Deli beef

Item	Quantity		Directions
Bread, white slice, store	2	Each	Makes 1 sandwich.
Mayonnaise, Light	1	Tablespoon	Spread evenly on both slices of bread.
Horseradish, prepared	1	Tablespoon	Spread evenly on one slice of bread.
Roast beef, deli style, sliced	6	Each	Place evenly on bread.
Lettuce, iceberg	1/2	Ounce	Place 1 large leaf on top of beef.
			Place second slice of bread on top of beef. Enjoy

Comments:

6 slices of beef is about 2 ounces. Notice the large amount of sodium and potassium in deli beef. Measure beef by weight.

Serving Size 160 grams About 5.6 oz. Recipe Total Weight About 5.6 oz.

Water	Calories	Protein	Fat	Carbs	Fiber	Sugars	Phos*	Pot*	Sodium*
99	269	16	8	34	2	6	204	499	964

* Values are in mg. All others are in grams

Roast Beef, home cooked

Item	Quantity		Directions
			Makes 1 sandwich.
Bread, Homemade, 1 slice	1	Each	Cut 1 slice of bread in half.
Mayonnaise, Light	1	Tablespoon	Spread evenly on both slices of bread.
Horseradish, prepared	1	Tablespoon	Spread evenly on one slice of bread.
Beef, Roast, homemade	2	Ounce	Slice very thin, Place evenly on bread.
Lettuce, iceberg	1/2	Ounce	About 1 large leaf; Place on top of beef.
			Place second slice of bread on top of beef; enjoy.

Comments:

Roast beef is high in phosphorous, potassium and sodium

Serving Size 159 grams About 5.6 oz. Recipe Total Weight About 5.6 oz.

Water	Calories	Protein	Fat	Carbs	Fiber	Sugars	Phos*	Pot*	Sodium*
100	289	16	12	29	2	3	165	305	395

* Values are in mg. All others are in grams

Tuna Salad

Item	Quantity		Directions
			Makes 8.1 ounces (230g); enough for 2 small sandwiches, or 1 large sandwich.
Tunafish in water (5 oz can)	1	Can	Place in small bowl.
Miracle Whip	2	Tablespoon	Add to bowl.
Onions,	2	Tablespoon	Dice; add to bowl.
Pickle, Bread & Butter	5	Each	Dice 5 slices; add to bowl; mix.
Pepper, Black ground	1/8	Teaspoon	Add to bowl, mix.

Comments:

115 grams is enough for 1 sandwich.

Serving Size 115 grams About 4.1 oz. Recipe Total Weight About 8.1 oz.

Water	Calories	Protein	Fat	Carbs	Fiber	Sugars	Phos*	Pot*	Sodium*
79	123	14	4	7	0	5	121	283	363

* Values are in mg. All others are in grams

Tuna Salad Sandwich

Item	Quantity		Directions
			Makes 1 sandwich, 6.2 ounces (176g) each.
Bread, white slice, store	2	Each	
Tuna Salad	106	Gram	Spread evenly on one slice of bread.
Lettuce, iceberg	10	Gram	Layer shredded lettuce on tuna salad.
			Cover with second piece of bread; cut in half.

Serving Size 174 grams About 6.1 oz. Recipe Total Weight About 6.2 oz.

Water	Calories	Protein	Fat	Carbs	Fiber	Sugars	Phos*	Pot*	Sodium*
103	271	18	6	36	2	8	171	348	622

* Values are in mg. All others are in grams

Tuna Sandwich

Item	Quantity		Directions
			Makes tuna for 2 sandwiches 3.9 ounces 110g) each
Tuna fish in water (5 oz can)	1	Can	Add to bowl, break apart.
Miracle Whip	1 1/4	Tablespoon	Add to small bowl and mix well.
Bread, white slice, store	4	Each	Spread half of tuna on one slice of bread,
			cover with 2nd slice of bread; cut in half.

Serving Size 141 grams About 5 oz. Recipe Total Weight About 9.9 oz.

Water	Calories	Protein	Fat	Carbs	Fiber	Sugars	Phos*	Pot*	Sodium*
78	247	19	5	31	2	4	168	279	534

* Values are in mg. All others are in grams

Seasonings

Chili Powder

Item	Quantity		Directions
			Makes about 1 ounce
Pepper, Red ground	2	Tablespoon	Add to small bowl
Cumin	1 1/2	Tablespoon	Add to bowl
Oregano	1	Tablespoon	Add to bowl
Garlic, Granulated	1	Tablespoon	Add to bowl, mix and put in spice jar

Serving Size 5 grams About 0.2 oz. Recipe Total Weight About 1.2 oz

Water	Calories	Protein	Fat	Carbs	Fiber	Sugars	Phos*	Pot*	Sodium*
0	16	1	1	3	1	0	18	83	16

* Values are in mg. All others are in grams

Italian Sausage Seasoning

Item	Quantity		Directions
			Makes enough for 16 pounds of medium hot sausage.
Pepper, Red ground	2	Tablespoon	Add to small bowl.
Pepper, Crushed red	2	Tablespoon	Add to bowl.
Pepper, Black ground	2	Tablespoon	Add to bowl.
Fennel seed	1/4	Cup	Add to bowl.
Basil, dried leaves	2	Tablespoon	Add to bowl.
Salt, table	1	Tablespoon	Add to bowl and mix well.
			Use 3/4 tablespoon of mix per pound of ground pork for medium hot sausage.

Comments:

Enough to make 16 pounds of Kidney friendly Italian Sausage ---3/4 table spoon is a serving size of 4.8 grams, --this makes 1 pound of medium hot sausage

Serving Size 5 grams About 0.2 oz. Recipe Total Weight 81 grams About 2.9 oz.

Water	Calories	Protein	Fat	Carbs	Fiber	Sugars	Phos*	Pot*	Sodium*
0	11	1	0	2	1	0	12	67	422

* Values are in mg. All others are in grams

Poultry Seasoning

Item	Quantity		Directions
Pepper, Black ground	2	Tablespoon	Add to small jar.
Sage, dry ground	2	Tablespoon	Add to jar.
Thyme, dried Leaves	2	Teaspoon	Add to jar.
Savory, ground	2	Teaspoon	Add to jar and shake well.
			Makes about 5 tablespoons of seasoning: 21g (.7 ounces).

Serving Size 5 grams About 0.2 oz. Recipe Total Weight About 0.8 oz.

Water	Calories	Protein	Fat	Carbs	Fiber	Sugars	Phos*	Pot*	Sodium*
1	13	1	0	3	2	0	8	60	1

* Values are in mg. All others are in grams

Sausage Seasoning, Breakfast; HI salt

Item	Quantity		Directions
			Makes enough for 3 pounds of pork. This is a **HIGH salt** recipe
Sage, dry ground	2	Tablespoon	Add to small bowl
Marjoram, dried	1/2	Tablespoon	Add to bowl
Salt, table	1	Tablespoon	Add to bowl
Pepper, Black ground	1	Tablespoon	Add to bowl
			Add to bowl, mix well, store in air tight jar
			Use 1 tsp of mix per 4 ounces of meat, or 4 tsp per 1 pound of meat.

Comments:

This is a high salt recipe and is not recommended for a kidney diet.

Serving Size 30 grams About 1.1 oz. Recipe Total Weight 30 grams About 1.1 oz.

Water	Calories	Protein	Fat	Carbs	Fiber	Sugars	Phos*	Pot*	Sodium*
5	125	5	3	30	15	1	70	606	27

* Values are in mg. All others are in grams

Sausage Seasoning, Breakfast; LOW salt

Item	Quantity		Directions
			Enough for 3 pounds of pork. This is a **Low salt** recipe.
Sage, dry ground	2	Tablespoon	Add to small bowl.
Marjoram, dried	1/2	Tablespoon	Add to bowl.
Salt, table	1	Teaspoon	Add to bowl.
Pepper, Black ground	1	Tablespoon	Add to bowl. Mix well, store in air tight jar.
			Use 4 teaspoons of mix for each pound of ground pork

Serving Size 18 grams About 0.6 oz. Recipe Total Weight 18 grams About 0.6 oz.

Water	Calories	Protein	Fat	Carbs	Fiber	Sugars	Phos*	Pot*	Sodium*
1	35	1	1	8	4	0	19	161	2,5

* Values are in mg. All others are in grams

Sausage Seasoning, Breakfast; Medium salt

Item	Quantity		Directions
			Enough for 3 pounds of pork. This is a medium salt recipe.
Sage, dry ground	2	Tablespoon	Add to small bowl.
Marjoram, dried	1/2	Tablespoon	Add to bowl.
Salt, table	2	Teaspoon	Add to bowl.
Pepper, Black ground	1	Tablespoon	Add to bowl. mix well, store in air tight jar.
			Use 4 teaspoons of mix for each pound of ground pork.

Comments:

This is a medium salt recipe and is not recommended for anyone on a kidney diet.

Serving Size 25 grams About 0.9 oz. Recipe Total Weight About 0.9 oz.

Water	Calories	Protein	Fat	Carbs	Fiber	Sugars	Phos*	Pot*	Sodium*
1	34	1	1	8	4	0	18	156	4,9

* Values are in mg. All others are in grams

About The Author

William has a degree in electronic engineering from Syracuse University and has been solving all manner of problems for his entire life.

During his spare time, he built a home, fixed whatever had broken, raised chickens, kept horses, and developed recipes. Whew! That's in addition to his full-time job of inventing all kinds of electronic things.

INDEX

Made in United States
Orlando, FL
04 November 2026

90202230R00096